Atrial Septal Defects

Atrial Septal Defects

Diagnosis and Management

Edited by

Dr Ajith Ananthakrishna Pillai

MD, DM, FRCP (London), FACC (USA), FSCAI (USA)
Senior Consultant Interventional Cardiology and
Structural Heart Program
Additional Professor of Cardiology, JIPMER, Puducherry, India

Dr Vidhyakar Balasubramanian

MD, DM (Cardiology), FSCAI (USA), PDF (Cardiac
Electrophysiology), CCDS (IBHRE, USA)
Assistant Professor and Consultant Cardiologist
PSGIMSR, Coimbatore, India

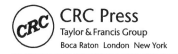

CRC Press
Taylor & Francis Group
Boca Raton London New York

CRC Press is an imprint of the
Taylor & Francis Group, an **informa** business

First edition published 2021
by CRC Press
6000 Broken Sound Parkway NW, Suite 300, Boca Raton, FL 33487-2742
and by CRC Press

2 Park Square, Milton Park, Abingdon, Oxon, OX14 4RN

© 2021 Taylor & Francis Group, LLC

CRC Press is an imprint of Taylor & Francis Group, LLC

Library of Congress Cataloging-in-Publication Data

Names: Pillai, Ajith Ananthakrishna, editor. | Balasubramanian, Vidhyakar, editor.
Title: Atrial septal defects : diagnosis and management / edited by Dr. Ajith Ananthakrishna Pillai, Dr. Vidhyakar Balasubramanian.
Description: First edition. | Boca Raton, FL : CRC Press, 2021. | Includes bibliographical references and index. | Summary: "This comprehensive text follows an evidence-based approach to thoroughly discuss Atrial septal defects. Since this congenital heart disease mostly presents in adulthood, it becomes imperative to understand the embryology, pathophysiology and anatomy in detail, for effective management of these patients. This book has strong clinical focus on anatomy, natural history, indications, imaging methods and practical aspects of disease management, which inculcates best practice in the day to day management techniques employed by cardiologists, trainees and professionals"– Provided by publisher.
Identifiers: LCCN 2020052676 (print) | LCCN 2020052677 (ebook) | ISBN 9780367568337 (paperback) | ISBN 9780367568351 (hardback) | ISBN 9781003099550 (ebook)
Subjects: MESH: Heart Septal Defects, Atrial–diagnostic imaging | Heart Septal Defects, Atrial–surgery | Echocardiography–methods | Cardiac Catheterization–methods
Classification: LCC RC683.5.U5 (print) | LCC RC683.5.U5 (ebook) | NLM WG 220 | DDC 616.1/207543–dc23
LC record available at https://lccn.loc.gov/2020052676
LC ebook record available at https://lccn.loc.gov/2020052677

ISBN: 9780367568351 (hbk)
ISBN: 9780367568337 (pbk)
ISBN: 9781003099550 (ebk)

Typeset in Minion Pro
by KnowledgeWorks Global Ltd.

Contents

Preface

When the idea of writing a comprehensive book on device closure of ostium secundum ASD came to us, we were confident in delivering the material as we had exposure to different aspects of interventional training in device closure of ASDs, PFOs, VSDs and PDAs in both adult and paediatric patients. The book is a comprehensive review of all the aspects of ostium secundum ASDs from anatomy, embryology, pathophysiology and imaging to various aspects of transcatheter device-closure techniques. Transcatheter closure of complex ASDs has been extensively reviewed in a separate chapter. Imaging of the septum and assessment of the rims which form an important decision-making step have been given immense importance, explaining in detail regarding transthoracic, transesophageal echocardiography of the atrial septal defect. Three-dimensional transthoracic and transesophageal echocardiography, along with intracardiac echocardiography, have been extensively dealt with in this book for better understanding of larger and complex ASDs during interventional device-closure procedure.

We hope that readers will enjoy reading this book and gain essential knowledge in their practice of device closure from practical tips given throughout this book.

Dr Ajith Ananthakrishna Pillai
Dr Vidhyakar Balasubramanian

Acknowledgements

Thanks to our patients who formed the basis of our experience and learning in this journey of interventions in congenital cardiac disease. I would like to express my gratitude to Dr Amit Handa, Dr Chandramohan and Dr Kabilan for their immense contributions in various chapters of this book. I would like to thank Miss Saranya Gousy for her wonderful illustrative diagrams throughout this book. I would like to thank Dr Vidhyakar Balasubramanian for co-editing this manuscript. We hope that the best outcome of this book is sharing of our vast experience and knowledge in the aspects of procedural decision-making which will be a great boon for practising interventional cardiologists and paediatric interventional cardiology practice.

I would like to thank Himani Dwivedi and Shivangi Pramanik of CRC Press/Taylor & Francis Group for their immense and valuable support for bringing out this manuscript, bearing all the delay during this difficult situation amidst a pandemic.

Dr Ajith Anathakrishna Pillai

About the editors

Dr Ajith Ananthakrishna Pillai is currently the head of the Department of Cardiology, JIPMER. He has mentored many students in the field of interventional cardiology over the past 12 years and has a vast experience in complex coronary interventions and nonsurgical management of congenital and structural heart diseases in both paediatric and adult populations. He is an interventional cardiologist of national repute and has represented as an international faculty in many interventional cardiology programs such as TCT, TCTAP and EURO PCR. He has authored more than 50 peer-reviewed journal articles and co-authored books on interventional cardiology. He is the driving force and lead author for this current project: *Atrial Septal Defects: Diagnosis and Management*.

Dr Vidhyakar Balasubramanian has worked as a senior resident and completed a DM residency program from the Department of Cardiology, JIPMER (2014). He completed a fellowship training programme in cardiac devices and electrophysiology at the prestigious Jayadeva Institute of Cardiology in 2017. He was certified as a specialist in cardiac devices (CCDS) by the Heart Rhythm Society in the US. He has been associated with the principal author, Dr Ajith Ananthakrishna Pillai, in various academic and research activities. He is currently working as an assistant professor in the Department of Cardiology, PSGIMSR, Coimbatore. He has co-authored many national and international journal articles.

Contributors

V Balasubramanian MD, DM, FSCAI, PDF, CCDS
PSGIMSR
Coimbatore, India

R Chandramohan MD, DM
Consultant Cardiologist
Royal Care Hospital
Coimbatore, India

Saranya Gousy BSc
Cath Lab Technologist
JIPMER
Pondicherry, India

A Handa MD, DM
Consultant Cardiologist
IVY Hospital
Hoshiarpur, Punjab, India

SJ Kabilan MD, DM
Department of Cardiology
JIPMER
Pondicherry, India

AA Pillai MD, DM, FRCP, FACC, FSCAI
JIPMER
Pondicherry, India

Classification and natural history

A A PILLAI, A HANDA, V BALASUBRAMANIAN, SARANYA GOUSY

INTRODUCTION

Atrial septal defects (ASDs) are common, constituting approximately 8–10% of congenital heart disorders, with a reported prevalence at birth of approximately 2 per 1000 live births. The clinical consequences of an ASD are related to the anatomic location of the defect, its size and the presence or absence of other cardiac anomalies.[1] ASDs may be related to mutations in regulatory genes or sarcomeric genes. Heterozygous mutations in NKX2.5 were first reported in families with ostium secundum ASD as autosomal dominant inheritance. Mutations in other transcription factors such as TBX5, GATA4, TBX 2.0 have also been reported. Although most ASDs occur sporadically, familial mode of inheritance has been reported. ASDs have been reported to occur along with cardiomyopathies and are also associated to occur with syndromes such as Noonan, Down, Williams and Ellis-van Crevald. In addition to above-mentioned genetic diseases, they are also associated with maternal and environmental risk factors such as diabetes, anticonvulsants, anti-inflammatory drugs, retinoids, smoking and alcohol. The risk of congenital heart disease in the offspring of women with ostium secundum ASD is higher.

CLASSIFICATION

The various types of ASDs are classified on their different anatomic locations and abnormal embryogenesis:

Secundum ASD
Primum ASD
Sinus venosus ASD
Coronary sinus ASD

Patent foramen ovale (PFO) is also an open communication between the right and left atria; however, PFO is not considered an ASD because no septal tissue is missing.

Secundum defects—Secundum defects constitute approximately 75% of all ASDs and occur twice as often in females as in males.[2–5] Familial recurrent rate has been estimated to be about 7–10%.[6,7] A comprehensive review reported an incidence of 564 per million live births. The true incidence of secundum ASD may be much higher as many ASDs are commonly undiagnosed in infancy and childhood and spontaneously resolve before detection.

Secundum ASDs are located typically within the fossa ovalis (remnant of the foramen ovale in

Right septal view   Frontal view

(a) Normal

Fossa ovalis

Endocardial cushion

(b) Secundum ASD — Defect

(c) Primum ASD — Defect

(d) Sinus venosus ASD — Defect

■ Septum primum
■ Septum secundum

Figure 1.1 **(a)** The normal atrial septum as well as various types of ASDs is shown. **(b)** Secundum ASD formed by the poor growth of the septum secundum or excessive absorption of the septum primum. **(c)** Primum ASD formed by the failure of the septum primum to fuse with the endocardial cushions. The fossa ovalis is normal. The frontal view of the primum ASD shows the caudal location of the ASD just above the endocardial cushions. **(d)** Sinus venosus ASD caused by the malposition of the insertion of the superior or inferior vena cava and is outside the area of the fossa ovalis. (Illustration by Saranya Gousy.)

the right atrium). This type of ASD can result from arrested growth of the secundum septum or excessive absorption of the primum septum (Figure 1.1). If the floor of the fossa ovalis is fenestrated, multiple defects can be seen. The defects can vary greatly in size, from less than 5 mm to greater than 20 mm.

Secundum ASDs may be associated with or continuous with other ASDs, such as a sinus venosus defect or a primum defect. Some patients with secundum ASD have functional mitral valve prolapse, perhaps related to a change in the left ventricular geometry associated with right ventricular volume overload.[8,9]

Primum defects—The primum type ASD develops if the septum primum does not fuse with the endocardial cushions, leaving a defect at the base of the interatrial septum that is usually large

(Figure 1.1). The primum type of ASDs accounts for about 15–20% of total ASDs. Primum ASDs are usually not isolated, being typically associated with atrioventricular (AV) canal defects that include anomalies of the AV valves and defects of the ventricular septum.

Sinus venosus defects—Sinus venosus ASDs account for approximately 5–10% of all septal defects. Sinus venosus ASDs are characterized by malposition of the insertion of the superior or inferior vena cava straddling the atrial septum (Figure 1.2). The defect in these interatrial communications is not in the area of fossa ovalis but lies at the opening of the overriding vein.

Superior sinus venosus defects—Also referred to as superior vena caval defects, these are located just caudal to the opening of the superior vena

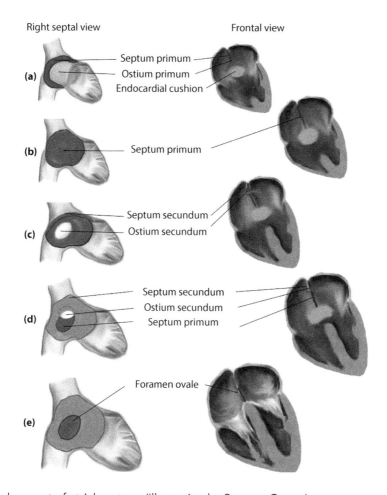

Right septal view   Frontal view

(a) Septum primum — Ostium primum — Endocardial cushion

(b) Septum primum

(c) Septum secundum — Ostium secundum

(d) Septum secundum — Ostium secundum — Septum primum

(e) Foramen ovale

Figure 1.2 Development of atrial septum. (Illustration by Saranya Gousy.)

cava (SVC). These defects are often associated with a partial anomalous pulmonary venous connection as the right upper and middle lobe pulmonary veins often connect to the junction of the SVC and right atrium, which results in a partial anomalous pulmonary venous connection.[10,11]

Inferior sinus venosus defects—Also referred to as inferior vena caval defects, these are comparatively less common. They are found immediately cranial to the orifice of the inferior vena cava. These defects are also often associated with partial anomalous connection of the right pulmonary veins.

Coronary sinus defects—In coronary sinus defects (unroofed coronary sinus), part of or the entire wall between the coronary sinus and the left atrium is absent. This form accounts for less than 1% of all ASDs. Many patients with coronary sinus ASDs may also have a persistent left superior vena cava.[12]

Patent foramen ovale—Approximately 30% of normal adult hearts have a PFO. Defects typically range from 1 to 10 mm in maximal potential diameter.[13] A PFO is usually not considered an ASD because no septal tissue is missing. Interatrial shunting cannot occur as long as left atrial pressure exceeds right atrial pressure and the flap valve remnant of septum primum of the foramen ovale is competent. However, persistent left-to-right shunting frequently occurs in the first few weeks of life. The presence of a mild degree of shunting during the neonatal period, particularly in premature infants, is so common that it is usually considered a normal variant finding.

Natural history of unoperated ASDs

Most of the patients with ostium secundum ASDs are asymptomatic except the larger ones. Smaller ostium secundum ASDs, especially those less than 5 mm, close spontaneously. They are mostly asymptomatic in childhood, coming to attention in second or third decade. They may present with abnormal auscultatory findings, especially of pulmonary overcirculation or abnormal ECG, echocardiograms or chest X-ray findings. They may also present to paediatrician with recurrent respiratory tract infections and very rarely with failure to thrive, and cyanosis on exertion may be due to development of pulmonary artery hypertension. They may present with exertional dyspnoea in older age due to comorbidities such as hypertension or coronary artery disease.[14] They may rarely present with atrial arrhythmias and rarely with transient ischaemic attacks or cerebrovascular accident. Campbell in 1970 reported negligible mortality in the first to second decades and later on increases to 2.7% in the third, 5.4% in fourth and fifth and 7.5% in sixth decade; median age of death was 37 years, and none survived to the eighth or ninth decade.[2] The increase in late mortality is mainly due to development of pulmonary vascular disease and development of Eisenmenger syndrome and right heart failure and atrial arrhythmias.

Natural history in the era of transcatheter closure

Closure of ostium secundum ASDs at any age has shown improvement in symptoms, right ventricular function and pulmonary artery pressure, but the best outcome was in patients with fewer symptoms and closure at younger age. Transcatheter closure of ASDs has changed the natural history of ASDs drastically. Patients with moderate to large ASDs benefit the most when they are closed before their second or third decade. The incidence of late onset arrhythmias, pulmonary artery hypertension and right heart failure is prevented and has drastically reduced mortality. The scenario is not same in the elderly age group, where the benefit of ASD closure is based on multiple comorbid factors. Smaller defects which are less than 3 mm close spontaneously or may become PFO. Larger defects, especially more than 12 mm, remain the same or may grow by 0.8 mm per year. The optimal device for closure and optimal timing is still a contentious issue. The natural history of large defects has not been studied extensively. But a lot of development has gone into transcatheter device technology, and for even largest of the defects device closure is attempted nowadays. Elective closure of moderate to large ASD is advised by 4–6 years of age. Two-thirds of large secundum ASDs enlarge in size and may outgrow transcatheter closure of select devices. Availability of larger devices may circumvent this problem.[15]

REFERENCES

1. Van der Linde D, Konings EE, Slager MA, et al. Birth prevalence of congenital heart disease worldwide: A systematic review and meta-analysis. *J Am Coll Cardiol*. 2011; 58:2241.
2. Campbell M. Natural history of atrial septal defect. *Br Heart J*. 1970; 32:820–26.
3. Gelernter-Yaniv L, Lorber A. The familial form of atrial septal defect. *Acta Paediatr*. 2007; 96:726.
4. Hoffman JI, Kaplan S. The incidence of congenital heart disease. *J Am Coll Cardiol*. 2002; 39:1890.
5. McMahon CJ, Feltes TF, Fraley JK, et al. Natural history of growth of secundum atrial septal defects and implications for trans catheter closure. *Heart*. 2002; 87:256.
6. Riggs T, Sharp SE, Batton D, et al. Spontaneous closure of atrial septal defects in premature vs. full-term neonates. *Pediatr Cardiol*. 2000; 21:129.
7. Helgason H, Jonsdottir G. Spontaneous closure of atrial septal defects. *Pediatr Cardiol*. 1999; 20:195.
8. Brassard M, Fouron JC, van Doesburg NH, et al. Outcome of children with atrial septal defect considered too small for surgical closure. *Am J Cardiol*. 1999; 83:1552–55.
9. Caputo S, Capozzi G, Russo MG, et al. Familial recurrence of congenital heart disease in patients with ostium secundum atrial septal defect. *Eur Heart J*. 2005; 26:2179.
10. Suchoń E, Podolec P, Płazak W, et al. Mitral valve prolapse associated with ostium secundum atrial septal defect—a functional disorder. *Acta Cardiol*. 2004; 59:237.

11. VanPraagh S, Geva T, Lock JE, et al. Biatrial or left atrial drainage of the right superior vena cava: Anatomic, morphogenetic, and surgical considerations—report of three new cases and literature review. *Pediatr Cardiol.* 2003; 24:350.

12. Raghib G, Ruttenberg HD, Anderson RC, Amplatz K, Adams P, Edwards JE. Termination of left superior vena cava in left atrium, atrial septal defect, and absence of coronary sinus: A developmental complex. *Circulation.* 1965; 31:906–18.

13. Joy J, Kartha CC, Balakrishnan KG. Structural basis for mitral valve dysfunction associated with ostium secundum atrial septal defects. *Cardiology.* 1993; 82:409.

14. Samianek M. Children with congenital heart disease: Probability of natural survival. *Pediatr Cardiol.* 1992; 13:152–8.

15. Therrien J, Webb G. Clinical update on adults with congenital heart disease. *Lancet.* 2003; 362:1305.

2

Pathophysiology

A A PILLAI, A HANDA, R CHANDRAMOHAN

The pathophysiology of isolated atrial septal defects (ASDs) depends upon the relationship of pulmonary and systemic resistances, the compliance of the right and left ventricles and the size of the defect.

Perinatal physiology—In utero, pulmonary arterial blood flow in the foetus is limited by high pulmonary vascular resistance. As a result, the blood that flows into the right atrium is shunted across the isolated ASD into the left atrium, similar to the blood flow through the normal patent foramen ovale. At birth, left atrial pressure becomes greater than right atrial pressure resulting in left-to-right shunting across the defect. Initially, the volume of blood shunted from left to right is small because the right ventricle is still relatively thick-walled and noncompliant. As the right ventricle remodels in response to the decreased pulmonary vascular resistance, its compliance increases and the mean right atrial pressure decreases. As a result, the left-to-right shunting increases in volume.

In some neonates, transient right-to-left shunting may also occur during the cardiac and respiratory cycles, resulting in mild cyanosis. In these patients, there is a drop in atrial pressure at the onset of ventricular contraction due to atrial relaxation that is more rapid in the left than the right atrium. During inspiration, the decrease in intrathoracic pressure results in an increase in systemic venous return and a decrease in pulmonary venous return, decreasing left atrial pressure and increasing right atrial pressure, which results in right-to-left shunting.

Postnatal physiology—Although there are several forms of ASDs, the pathophysiology is similar. With a small ASD, left atrial pressure is slightly higher than right atrial pressure, resulting in continuous flow of oxygenated blood from the left to the right atrium across the defect. The pressure gradient between the two atria and the amount of shunt flow depends upon the size of the defect and the relative distensibility of the right and left sides of the heart. Left-to-right shunting occurs primarily in the late ventricular systole and early diastole and with augmentation during atrial systole. Even when the right and left atrial pressures are equal, as will be seen with a large defect, left-to-right shunting still occurs because of the greater compliance of the right ventricle compared with the left ventricle.

The shunt flow constitutes a circuit through the right atrium, right ventricle, pulmonary circulation, left atrium and defects back to the right atrium. Thus, the volume of blood flow in the pulmonary circulation is greater than that in the systemic circulation.

The increased flow leads to right-sided dilatation, evident on chest radiograph and echocardiographic imaging. Right ventricular function is also occasionally decreased. The main pulmonary arteries dilate and the pulmonary vascularity is increased. These pulmonary vascular changes may be evident on the chest radiograph, and large vessels in both the lower and upper lobes may be seen.

Heart failure is unusual before the age of 30, but the prevalence increases substantially in older uncorrected patients over time; right-sided volume overload is usually well tolerated for years.

Other complications in older patients include atrial arrhythmias such as flutter and fibrillation, thought to result from chronic stretching of the atrial muscle, and occasionally, pulmonary arteriopathy leading to progressive pulmonary hypertension resulting in right-to-left shunting of blood (i.e., Eisenmenger syndrome).

NATURAL HISTORY

The natural course of isolated ASDs, which are primarily secundum ASDs, varies from spontaneous closure to enlarging defects and increasing symptoms.

Spontaneous closure—Spontaneous closure, or a decrease in size, is most likely to occur in younger patients and those with defects less than 7–8 mm in diameter.[1]

In a review of 101 infants diagnosed at a mean age of 26 days and with an average follow-up of 9 months, spontaneous closure occurred in all 32 patients with ASDs <3 mm in diameter, 87% of patients with 3–5 mm ASDs, 80% of patients with 5–8 mm ASDs and in none of the four infants with defects larger than 8 mm.[2]

In a study of 200 children diagnosed at a mean age of 5 months (range 0.1 months to 13.9 years) who were followed up at a mean of 3.5 years[3] (range 0.5–9.4 years), spontaneous closure or a decrease in size <3 mm in diameter was observed in 69 of 81 patients (85%) with 4–5 mm ASDs, in 36 of 56 patients (64%) with 6–7 mm ASDs and in 15 of 41 patients (36%) with 8–10 mm ASDs; in 22 patients with an ASD >10 mm, there was no spontaneous resolution, but two had a defect that regressed to <3 mm. Children less than 1 year of age compared with older children were more likely to experience spontaneous resolution (39 versus 19%).[4] Surgical or transcatheter closure was required in 11, 32 and 77% of patients with defects of 4–5 mm, 6–7 mm, and >10 mm, respectively.

Persistent moderate to large ASDs—In patients with uncorrected moderate to large ASDs, left-to-right shunting may increase with age. As a result, the frequency of heart failure accompanied by fluid retention, hepatomegaly and elevated jugular venous pressure increases with advancing age. Most such patients become symptomatic before 40 years of age. Common symptoms are palpitations, which reflect atrial arrhythmias (the most frequent presenting symptom of ASDs), exercise intolerance, dyspnoea and fatigue. Arrhythmias are thought to result from stretching of the atria by the increased shunting. In some patients, exercise intolerance may develop as early as the second decade of life.

The right-sided volume overload associated with an ASD is usually well tolerated for years. Pulmonary vascular disease develops in about 10% of older patients with isolated ASDs, but this complication is rare in childhood and adolescence. In a retrospective study over a 10-year period from two tertiary centres, only 8 of 355 paediatric patients (2%) with isolated ASDs had severe pulmonary hypertension.[5] These eight infants (six with secundum and two with primum ASDs) had elevated pulmonary arterial pressures (PAP) of 50–100% of systemic pressure and were operated on within the first year of life with subsequent normalization of PAP. These results highlight that elevated pulmonary vascular resistance in infants with ASDs is almost always reversible with correction, unlike the rare complication of fixed pulmonary vascular disease seen in affected adults.

In uncorrected older patients, severe irreversible pulmonary hypertension (Eisenmenger syndrome) may develop and presents with signs of right ventricular failure resulting in right-to-left shunting.[5] Clinical findings include cyanosis, dyspnoea with exertion, hepatomegaly and clubbing of the fingers and toes. These patients are also at risk for paradoxical embolization of clot from the venous system or right atrium via right-to-left shunting into the arterial system.

CLINICAL FEATURES

Presentation

Primum ASD—Prenatal ultrasounds can usually diagnose primum ASDs in the foetus at 18–22 weeks' gestation.

Secundum ASD—The more common secundum ASDs cannot be reliably detected by fetal echocardiography, since the normal foetus has a sizeable patent foramen ovale, and distinguishing between a small to moderate size secundum ASD and a patent foramen ovale with right-to-left flow is usually not possible. However, the presence of very large secundum ASDs may be suspected on fetal echocardiography, but must be confirmed by postnatal echocardiograms.

Sinus venosus and coronary sinus ASDs— Fetal echocardiographers may be able to detect sinus venosus ASDs and coronary sinus ASDs. However, the sensitivity and specificity of fetal ultrasound for identification of these more unusual types of ASD is not known.

Postnatal—The apparent incidence of ASDs may be increasing because of increased usage of echocardiography in the neonatal period. Many secundum ASDs or incompetent foramen ovales identified on echocardiograms obtained for nonspecific indications in early infancy will close spontaneously during later infancy or early childhood.

Because most ASDs are small and do not cause symptoms in infancy and childhood, many postnatal presentations occur during a routine physical examination when a cardiac murmur is detected incidentally. In one large case series of 481 patients with an ASD who were seen between 1957 and 1976, and who underwent corrective surgery before the age of 40, ASD was identified during routine examination in 202 (42%).[6]

Infants with large ASDs may present with heart failure, recurrent respiratory infections or failure to thrive.[7] Failure to thrive in infants with ASDs may be associated with extracardiac pathology.[8] Migraine headaches, particularly migraine headaches with auras, have been associated with ASDs in observational studies. However, the relationship between ASDs and migraines remains controversial, since a causal relationship has not been demonstrated by randomized trials.

Paradoxical embolization and resultant embolic stroke can, of course, occur through an ASD or patent foramen ovale. However, strokes are rare in paediatric patients, and there is no evidence at the present time that pre-emptive ASD or patent foramen ovale closure or anticoagulant therapy in asymptomatic patients can prevent strokes.

In patients with uncorrected moderate to large ASDs, left-to-right shunting increases with age. Those with a significant flow across large ASDs (i.e., pulmonary to systemic flow more than 2:1) are likely to become symptomatic before the age of 40 years. Common symptoms include atrial arrhythmias (the most frequent presenting symptom), exercise intolerance, dyspnoea and fatigue. As the pulmonary blood flow increases, the pulmonary artery, capillaries and veins are dilated and lead to pulmonary flow-related hypertension. As the right atrium and ventricle are compliant, they dilate and lead to increase in left-to-right shunt and further increase in pulmonary blood flow. Long-standing increased pulmonary blood flow leads to medial hypertrophy of pulmonary arterioles and muscularization leading to pulmonary vascular occlusive disease, in turn leading to Eisenmenger syndrome when patient develops cyanosis initially on exertion then at rest.

REFERENCES

1. Lu J-H, Hsu T-L, Hwang B, Weng Z-C. Visualization of secundum atrial septal defect using transthoracic three-dimensional echocardiography in children: Implications for trans catheter closure. *Echocardiography*. 1998; 15: 651–60.

2. Attaran RR, Ata I, Kudithipudi V, Foster L, Sorrell VL. Protocol for optimal detection and exclusion of a patent foramen ovale using trans thoracic echocardiography with agitated saline microbubbles. *Echocardiography*. 2006; 23(7):616–22.

3. Lange A, Walayat M, Turnbull CM, et al. Assessment of atrial septal defect morphology by transthoracic three dimensional echocardiography using standard grey scale and Doppler myocardial imaging techniques: Comparison with magnetic resonance imaging and intraoperative findings. *Heart*. 1997; 78:382–9.

4. Konstantinides S, Kasper W, Geibel A, Hofmann T, Koster W, Just H. Detection of left-to-right shunting atrial septal defect by negative contrast echocardiography: A comparison of transthoracic and transesophageal approach. *Am Heart J*. 1993; 126:909–17.

5. Monte I, Grasso S, Licciardi S, Badano LP. Head-to-head comparison of real-time three-dimensional transthoracic echocardiography with transthoracic and

transesophageal two-dimensional contrast echocardiography for the detection of patent foramen ovale. *Eur J Echocardiogr.* 2010; 11:245–9.

6. Daniels C, Weytjens C, Cosyns B, et al. Second harmonic transthoracic echocardiography: The new reference screening method for the detection of patent foramen ovale. *Eur J Echocardiogr.* 2004; 5:449–52.

7. Mesihovic-Dinarevic S, Begic Z, Halimic M, Kadic A, Gojak R. The reliability of transthoracic and transesophageal echocardiography in predicting the size of atrial septal defect. *Acta Med Acad.* 2012; 41:145–53.

8. Mehta RH, Helmcke F, Nanda NC, Pinheiro L, Samdarshi TE, Shah VK. Uses and limitations of transthoracic echocardiography in the assessment of atrial septal defect in the adult. *Am J Cardiol.* 1991; 67:288–94.

3

Embryology and anatomy

A A PILLAI, A HANDA, V BALASUBRAMANIAN, SARANYA GOUSY

In the embryonic heart, the normal atrial septum, along with the surrounding atrial structures, is formed from several embryological tissue components that develop, remodel and fuse in the correct sequence. The development of the atrial septum occurs following the initial looping of the heart.

As the initial step in septation, a ridge of tissue develops from the superior aspect of the primary atrial component of the heart tube. This ridge is the primary septum (septum primum), and its leading edge is covered by cushion-like mesenchymal tissue that is continuous over the dorsal mesocardium. This dividing crest of tissue is part of the atrial chamber expressing genes demonstrating morphologically leftness.[1] As the atrial septum grows into the cavity, it extends down towards the endocardial cushions which are developing concomitantly within the atrioventricular (AV) canal. Normal septal development also involves incorporation of another mass of tissue derived from the dorsal mesocardium, known as the vestibular spine (spina vestibuli), and it, too, carries on its leading edge a mesenchymal cap. As the primary septum approaches the atrioventricular endocardial cushions, the various mesenchymal structures fuse together.[2] The spina vestibuli then muscularises, eventually forming the prominent infero-anterior border of the oval foramen. During the process of development the ventricular septum also 'moves' up towards the endocardial cushions, resulting in the septation of the ventricular chambers.[3]

Subsequent to the fusion between the primary septum and the endocardial cushions of the atrioventricular canal, the upper part of the primary septum disintegrates to form the ostium secundum. The remaining part of the primary septum becomes the flap valve of the fossa ovalis. The flap valve of the fossa ovalis, along with the muscularized antero-inferior rim, forms the true septum that separates the cavities of the atrial chambers. Only after integration of the pulmonary veins into the left atrium, the superior walls of the two atriums 'infold', creating the septum secundum in the superior portion of the atriums.[2] The flap valve overlaps, but is not completely adherent to, the rims of this superior atrial fold, known as the Waterston's or Sondergaard's groove, providing a passage for blood to pass from the right to the left atrium during foetal life (Figure 3.1). In postnatal life, this deep superior interatrial fold becomes filled with extracardiac fibro-fatty tissue[2] (Figure 3.2).

THE NORMAL POSTNATAL HEART

The atrial septum is best defined as the tissue which directly separates the atrial cavities, and which can be removed without excising walls or valves of the heart. When viewed in the light of this definition, the septum is confined to the thin flap of fibromuscular valvar tissue which forms the floor of the oval fossa, along with the immediate

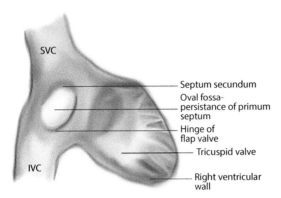

Septum secundum
Oval fossa-
persistance of primum
septum
Hinge of
flap valve
Tricuspid valve
Right ventricular
wall

SVC

IVC

Figure 3.1 Diagrammatic representation viewing the oval fossa from the right atrial aspect. The oval fossa flap valve and the immediate rim is the true extent of the atrial septum. (Illustration by Saranya Gousy.)

infero-anterior muscular rims of the fossa derived from the vestibular spine (Figure 3.3).

Thus, the septal area is only a small part of the wall dividing the atriums. The aortic mound, in contrast, which is to the right of the oval fossa when observed from the right atrial aspect, and which seems to represent an apparently solid muscular structure, is part of the external wall of the heart. Passage of an instrument through this area does not take one into the left atrium but rather into the transverse sinus of the pericardial cavity,

in front of the bulging right coronary sinus at the base of the aortic root (Figure 3.4). Similarly, passing a needle from the right to the left atrial chambers superiorly to the oval fossa also passes through extracardiac tissue, as this part of the dividing wall is in reality an infolding of the right atrial wall and hence is not septal (Figure 3.5). In adult life, this fold is filled with fatty extracardiac tissue. It is within this area that the sinus nodal artery usually takes its course (Figure 3.6). Morphologically, the distinct rims of the oval fossa are related to other important structures within the atrium. These can be viewed echocardiographically. The superior margin extends from the superior edge of the ASD towards the attachment of the superior caval vein within the right atrium. This superior rim is essentially an infolding of the muscular atrial walls. Progressing towards the postero-inferior rim of the defect, there is attachment of the inferior caval vein within the right atrium. The remaining border is the important anterior margin. This separates the margin of the oval fossa from the annulus of the tricuspid valve and the orifice of the coronary sinus (Figure 3.7). Full interrogation of the nature of these muscular borders of the oval fossa is crucial when assessing whether an interventional device can safely be fitted to close off a defect.

'Patent oval fossa and secundum defects within the fossa' are 'defects within the confines of the atrial septum'. In one-quarter to one-third of the

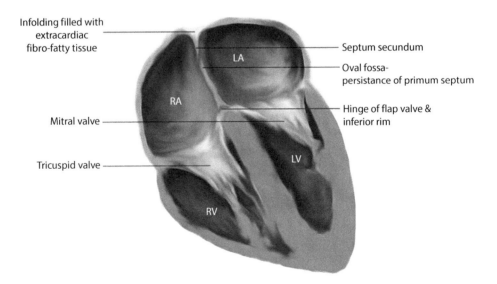

Infolding filled with extracardiac fibro-fatty tissue

Septum secundum
Oval fossa-
persistance of primum septum

LA

RA

Hinge of flap valve & inferior rim

Mitral valve

Tricuspid valve

LV

RV

Figure 3.2 Diagrammatic representation of the heart in four-chamber section. The flap valve overlaps the superiorly infolded walls of the atriums, partitioning the two chambers. (Illustration by Saranya Gousy.)

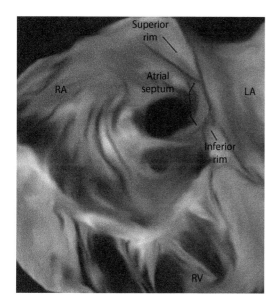

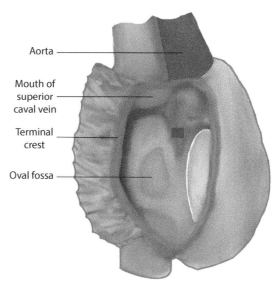

Figure 3.3 Four-chamber view of the RA and RV, showing the muscular superior and inferior rims and the flap valve of the oval fossa dividing the two atriums. (Illustration by Saranya Gousy.)

Figure 3.4 (a): Anterior view of the right atrium, showing the relationship of the aortic mound (red square) to the oval fossa.

normal population, the atrial septum does not close completely in the neonatal period. In these cases, the upper margin of the flap valve overlaps the infolded antero-superior rim of the oval fossa but does not become fused to it. Because of the failure of fusion, should right atrial pressure be higher than left, there is the potential for communication between the atriums within the region of the oval fossa. It is not due to any deficiency of the intrinsic septal structures, but it is created by a failure of the flap valve fully to adhere to the entirety of the rim. This lack of adhesion will permit a probe to be passed obliquely from the right to the left atrium. Usually probe patency is not physiologically significant, and it is often an incidental finding at post-mortem. The patent flap valve will permit interatrial shunting only occur when right atrial systemic pressure is higher than that in the left atrium.

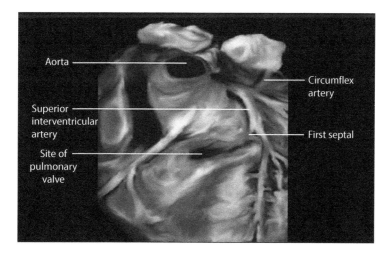

Figure 3.4 (b): A needle passing through the aortic mound (red square) would exit the heart into the transverse sinus. (Illustration by Saranya Gousy.)

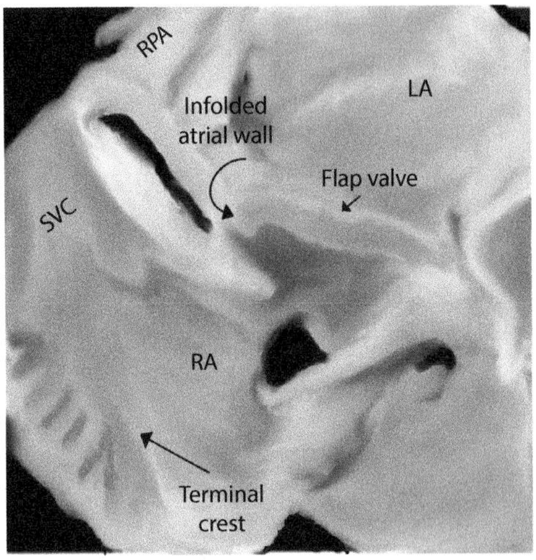

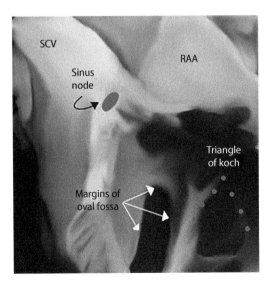

Figure 3.5 Four-chamber view showing the infolded right atrial wall, Waterston's groove, which is filled with extracardiac fat. (Illustration by Saranya Gousy.)

True defects of the atrial septum, of necessity confined within the bounds of the oval fossa, are often referred to as 'secundum' defects. The defect is a deficiency of the floor of the oval fossa, and this floor is derived from the primary atrial septum. Thus, the defects are 'ostium secundum' defects, and not deficiencies of the secondary atrial septum; the secondary 'septum' is no more than an infolding

Figure 3.6 Anterior view showing the junction between the RAA and the SCV. This is the location of the sinus node and artery. (Illustration by Saranya Gousy.)

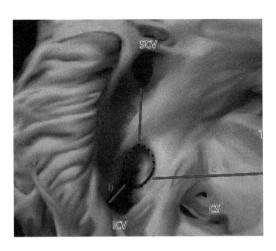

Figure 3.7 Right atrial view showing the oval fossa (black dots) surrounded by septal margins. (Illustration by Saranya Gousy.)

of the atrial roof. Such defects within the confines of the fossa account for over three-quarters of all defects between the atriums. In a study of 160 480 live births, ASDs were found to account for one-twentieth of all cases of congenital heart disease diagnosed in infancy.[3] The occurrence of congenital heart disease from various studies was reviewed, and overall incidence of ASDs was found to be 3.4/10 000 of all live births; and in adults with a congenital heart defect, ASDs comprise nearly one-third of all cases.[4]

There is a high probability of spontaneous closure of an isolated ASD in patients below the age of 5 years, with closure commonly occurring in up to 80% of the small-to-moderate-sized defects.[5] In one study, spontaneous closure was found in up to 60% of the population studied after the age of one and a half years, and about 40% of all patients after the age of 5 years.[6] The mechanism of spontaneous closure is not well known. Small ASDs can remain completely asymptomatic and hemodynamically insignificant throughout life.

Morphologically, there are notable variations in the structure of these ASDs. The differences impact on transcatheter closure. Intervention may not be possible if the defect is too large, or if there is a lack of suitable rims around the entire circumference to provide anchorage for a device. Other contraindications include the defect being displaced towards the posterior wall and its proximity to the entrance of the superior or inferior caval veins. Also, if the Eustachian valve is thick, this structure can obscure the postero-inferior rim of the oval fossa.

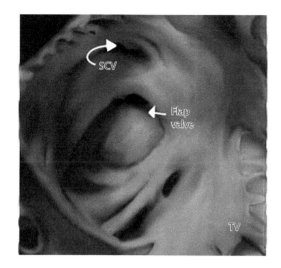

Figure 3.8 Right atrial view showing flap valve tissue that fails to fully cover the margins of the oval fossa. (Illustration by Saranya Gousy.)

When examined morphologically, seven-tenths of defects were centrally located defect within the confines of the oval fossa. Even within a group having these characteristics, the borders of the defect in two-fifths of the cases were deemed insufficient to provide firm anchorage for an occluding device.

The extent of deficiency of the flap valve can produce a spectrum of morphologies, ranging from the flap valve failing to cover the oval fossa completely (Figure 3.8) to its complete absence (Figure 3.9).

Absence of the flap valve, along with effacement of the rim, leads to a physiologically functional *common atrium*.

The floor morphology also varies, with some flap valves being very thin and membranous, composed of connective tissues, and others having integration of myocardium and so becoming thick and muscular.[7] This certainly has practical ramifications, such as performing the Rashkind procedure for atrial septostomy becomes much more difficult if a thicker and more muscular floor of the oval fossa is encountered. Once the defect is assessed, and it is determined that closure by device is recommended, then in ideal cases, this is a relatively straightforward procedure. Contraindications to closure include a large defect, even when a suitably large device is available. If the defect is unduly large, the device is likely to be adjacent to important structures with the atriums. The final position of the device is also of crucial importance, irrespective of the size of the defect, as its edges could impinge inferiorly in the right atrium on the coronary sinus, the atrioventricular nodal area and the inferior caval vein (Figure 3.10), or the device could encroach on the leaflets of the mitral valve in the left atrium. In one study, in about 33% of cases the narrowest boarder of the defect was between the oval fossa and the aortic mound, at the antero-superior rim. The same study showed

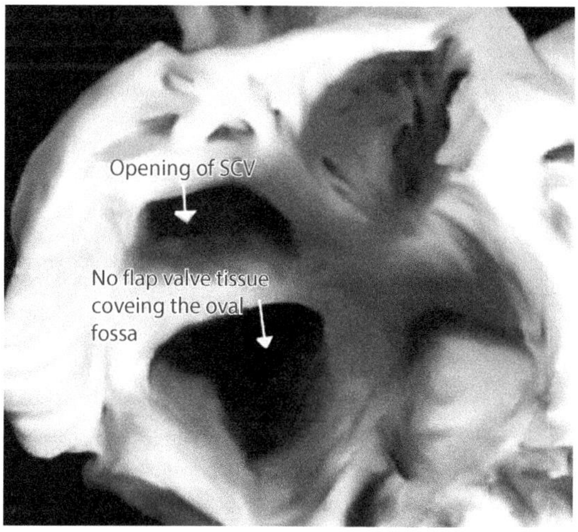

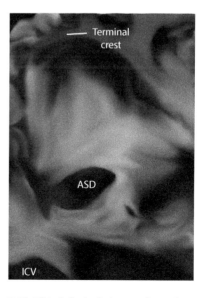

Figure 3.9 Right atrial view showing complete absence of the flap valve tissue. (Illustration by Saranya Gousy.)

Figure 3.10 This inferiorly located atrial septal defect is near the entrance of the ICV into the right atrium. (Illustration by Saranya Gousy.)

the superior rim to be furthest from the defect. A short rim in this position could result in the right upper and lower pulmonary veins being occluded on the left atrial aspect or the superior caval vein being obscured on the right atrial aspect.

REFERENCES

1. Oto A, Aytemir K, Ozkutlu S, et al. Transthoracic echocardiography guidance during percutaneous closure of patent foramen ovale. *Echocardiography*. 2011; 28:1074–80.
2. Siostrzonek P, Zangeneh M, Gössinger H, et al. Comparison of transesophageal and transthoracic contrast echocardiography for detection of a patent foramen ovale. *Am J Cardiol*. 1991; 68:1247–9.
3. Kronzon I, Tunick PA, Freedberg RS, Trehan N, Rosenzweig BP, Schwinger ME. Transesophageal echocardiography is superior to transthoracic echocardiography in the diagnosis of sinus venosus atrial septal defect. *J Am Coll Cardiol*. 1991; 17:537–42.
4. Zhu W, Cao QL, Rhodes J, Hijazi ZM. Measurement of atrial septal defect size: A comparative study between three-dimensional transesophageal echocardiography and the standard balloon sizing methods. *Pediatr Cardiol*. 2000; 21:465–9.
5. Belohlavek M, Foley DA, Gerber TC, Greenleaf JF, Seward JB. Three-dimensional ultrasound imaging of the atrial septum: Normal and pathologic anatomy. *J Am Coll Cardiol*. 1993; 22:1673–8.
6. Tobis J, Shenoda M. Percutaneous treatment of patent foramen ovale and atrial septal defects. *J Am Coll Cardiol*. 2012; 60:1722–32.
7. Zaqout M, Suys B, De Wilde H, De Wolf D. Transthoracic echocardiography guidance of trans catheter atrial septal defect closure in children. *Pediatr Cardiol*. 2009; 30:992–4.

4

Principles of imaging

A HANDA, SARANYA GOUSY

The evaluation of the abnormalities of interatrial septum (IAS) and its associated conditions and abnormalities require a standardized and systematic approach with echocardiographic and Doppler finding and characteristics, including transthoracic echocardiographic (TTE), transesophageal echocardiographic (TEE), intracardiac echocardiographic (ICE) ultrasound, three-dimensional (3D) imaging, Doppler and transcranial Doppler (TCD) modalities as and when indicated.

A thorough echocardiographic evaluation includes the detection and quantification of the size and shape of the septal defects, the rims of tissue surrounding the defect, the degree and direction of shunting and the remodelling and changes in size and function of the cardiac chambers and pulmonary circulation. The advent of 3D visualization, especially coupled with the transesophageal echocardiographic-based characterization, has contributed decisive incremental information in the evaluation of the IAS.

GENERAL IMAGING APPROACH

The most widely used modality for evaluation of the IAS is TTE, which is also the preferred initial diagnostic modality for the detection and diagnosis of patent foramen ovale (PFO), ASD and atrial septal aneurysm.[1] TTE is especially useful in small children in whom the ultrasound image quality will typically permit a full diagnostic study.[2] It can also be used for patient selection and real-time transcatheter ASD or PFO closure procedural guidance in paediatric patients.[4]

TTE can be used for the initial evaluation of ASD and PFO in adults; however, TEE is required to further characterize the atrial septal abnormalities, because the TTE image quality might not always permit a comprehensive evaluation of the IAS. TEE is not invariably required for assessment of a PFO if transcatheter closure is not being considered.[3] Also, 2D and 3D TEE offer significant incremental anatomic information compared with TTE and should be performed in all adult patients being evaluated for percutaneous transcatheter closure or surgical therapy.[3] In adults, TEE can identify the margins or rims of the ASD and assess the surrounding structures (e.g., aorta, cavae, pulmonary veins, AV valves and coronary sinus).

ICE is also used extensively to guide percutaneous ASD/PFO closure procedures and provides comparable but not identical imaging to TEE.[4]

Contrast echocardiography with agitated saline plays an important role in the evaluation of PFO and assessing residual shunts after transcatheter closure and has a more limited role in the diagnosis of ASD.[5]

Table 4.1 summarizes the recommended general imaging approach for atrial septal abnormalities stratified by the patient characteristics, imaging modality and intended application (e.g., diagnosis, procedure selection or guidance, follow-up).

THREE-DIMENSIONAL IMAGING OF THE INTERATRIAL SEPTUM

Three-dimensional TEE is described to improve the visualization of PFO and ASD, their surrounding tissue rims and surrounding structures and can also be used for guidance during percutaneous transcatheter closure.[3] IAS is a complex, dynamic and 3D anatomic structure; limitations exist in its evaluation using any single form of 2D echocardiography. The interatrial atrial septum and its associated abnormalities (such as ASD or PFO) do not exist in a true flat plane that can be easily aligned and interrogated using 2D imaging.[3] Both ASD and PFO exist in a wide variety of heterogeneous sizes, shapes and configurations (Figures 4.1 and 4.2). Three-dimensional imaging provides unique views of the IAS and, in particular, allows for en face viewing of the ASD and surrounding fossa, allowing for accurate determination of the ASD size and shape.[6] Furthermore, 3D imaging offers the potential to clearly and comprehensively define the dynamic morphology of the defect, which has been shown to change during the cardiac cycle. Also, 3D imaging delineates the relationship of the ASD to the surrounding cardiac structures and the rims of tissue surrounding it[2] (Figure 4.3).

Two-dimensional biplane (or triplane) imaging, a feature of currently commercially available 3D imaging systems, is a unique modality that takes advantage of 3D technology. The advantages of biplane imaging include the display of simultaneous additional echocardiographic views, with high frame rates and excellent temporal resolution.

Table 4.1 Imaging strategy for evaluation of atrial septal abnormalities[4]

Patient population	Establishing diagnosis of ASD or PFO	Imaging for transcatheter procedure	Routine post-procedure follow-up study
Paediatric patients <35–40 kg	TTE or TEE[a]	TEE or ICE[b]	TTE
Paediatric patients >35–40 kg	TTE, TEE or 3D TEE	TEE, 3D TEE or ICE	TTE
Adult patients	TTE, TEE or 3D TEE	TEE, 3D TEE or ICE	TTE

[a] Depending on body surface area and adequacy of image quality, TEE is recommended for assessment of an ASD; if the weight is >35–40 kg, 3D TEE can be performed.

[b] Use of ICE varies widely, some use ICE for procedure guidance of all defects; others use ICE for uncomplicated small ASD closure only, reserving TEE or 3D TEE for complicated or larger septal defects.

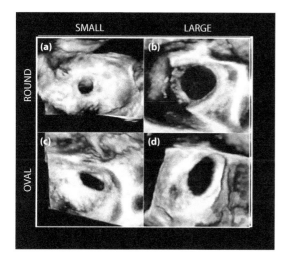

Figure 4.1 Three-dimensional transesophageal images of various shapes and sizes of ostium secundum ASD. Representative examples of round, small (a); round, large (b); oval, small (c); and oval, large (d) secundum ASD. (Adapted from ASE guidelines for echocardiographic assessment of ASD and PFO, August 2015.)

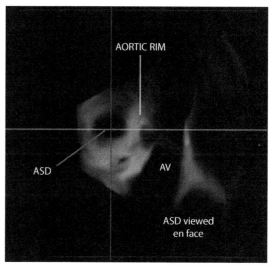

Figure 4.3 Three-dimensional ASD assessment allows for delineation of an ASD (blue arrow) and its relationship between adjacent structures. The aortic valve is seen, and the entire aortic rim (white arrow) is visualized en face. (Adapted from ASE guidelines for echocardiographic assessment of ASD and PFO, August 2015.)

Complementary simultaneously displayed orthogonal plane imaging provides incremental information compared with that from a single plane, and this imaging modality is uniquely suited to transcatheter procedure guidance. Numerous reports of the advantages of 3D TEE in guiding catheter interventions have been published and include the use of biplane imaging. Figure 4.4 illustrates the use of biplane imaging during percutaneous transcatheter closure of ASD before deployment of the device.

Also, 3D imaging allows for multiple acquisition modes, including narrow-angle, zoomed and wide-angle gated acquisition of multiple volumes. Once 3D volumes are acquired, post-processing using commercially available 3D software packages or 4D Cardio-View is performed to align the plane of the IAS with multiple 3D plane slices. This approach facilitates an assessment of the shape of an ASD and allows for measurement of the en face diameters in multiple orthogonal views, without the potential for bias due to malalignment of the ultrasound planes. The three-dimensional images should be reviewed in both systole and diastole to assess the dynamic changes in size which can occur. This 3D en face display can also aid in the recognition and quantification of rim deficiencies,

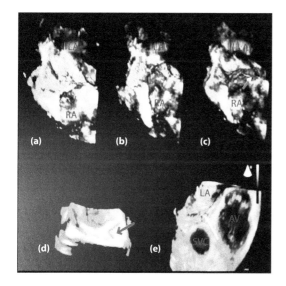

Figure 4.2 Three-dimensional TEE images of a PFO. Excessive movement of the septum primum (fossa ovalis) in a patient with an ASA and a PFO; red arrow white white arrow head specifies a PFO opened fully under influence of pressure difference between RA and LA (a–c). PFO 'tunnel' as viewed from the LA perspective; red arrow specifies the PFO exit into the LA (d). PFO tunnel exiting into LA (white arrow) (e). (Adapted from ASE guidelines for echocardiographic assessment of ASD and PFO, August 2015.)

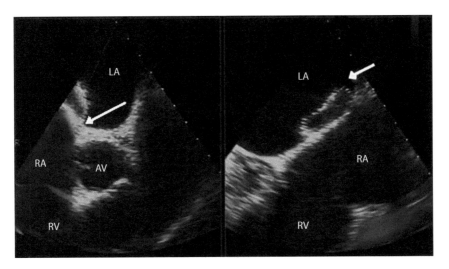

Figure 4.4 Biplane imaging performed during percutaneous transcatheter closure imaging of multiple planes simultaneously. The aortic rim and superior rim are seen (left arrow) and the device interaction with the aorta (left arrow) and atrial roof (right arrow) can be assessed simultaneously. (Adapted from ASE guidelines for echocardiographic assessment of ASD and PFO, August 2015.)

because the extent of the deficiency relative to the surrounding structures such as the aorta can be easily demonstrated and quantified. The distance between the defect and the aorta can be easily measured, just as can the area of the defect and length of rim deficiency when present.

ROLE OF ECHOCARDIOGRAPHY IN PERCUTANEOUS TRANSCATHETER DEVICE CLOSURE

The role of TTE, TEE and ICE during the assessment and transcatheter management of ASD/PFO is essential for appropriate patient selection, real-time procedure guidance, assessment of device efficacy and complications and long-term follow-up.[6] TTE provides information about the type of defect, its hemodynamic significance and any associated anomalies and can be used comprehensively in smaller paediatric patients for the diagnosis of ASD and PFO and even for patient selection and procedural guidance.[6] TTE has the advantage of offering unlimited multiple planes to evaluate the atrial septum, but it has limited ability to interrogate the lower rim of atrial septal tissue above the IVC after device placement, the device shadowing has an impact and interferes with imaging in almost all planes. In addition, because the septum is relatively far from the transducer, the image quality is often suboptimal in larger

paediatric and adult patients. If percutaneous closure is clinically indicated, a detailed assessment of the IAS anatomy and surrounding structures using TEE is typically required for patient selection and procedure guidance or ICE for procedure guidance in such patients. Transesophageal echocardiography provides real-time, highly detailed imaging of the IAS, surrounding structures, catheters and closure device during transcatheter closure. It requires either conscious sedation, with the attendant aspiration risk in a supine patient, or general anaesthesia, with an endotracheal tube placed to minimize aspiration risk. This approach also requires a dedicated echocardiographer to perform the TEE, while the interventionalist performs the transcatheter closure procedure. The advent of 3D TEE has enhanced the evaluation of ASD and PFO by clearly defining the IAS anatomy and enables an en face view of the defect and its surrounding structures.[7] Multiplesesreconstruction of the 3D data set allows accurate measurement of the minimum and maximum dimensions of the defect or defects, facilitating selection of the optimal size and type of closure device.[6] Moreover, intraprocedural real-time 3D TEE provides superior visualization of wires, catheters and devices and their relationships to neighbouring structures in a format that is generally more intuitively comprehended by the interventional cardiologist[8] (Figure 4.5).

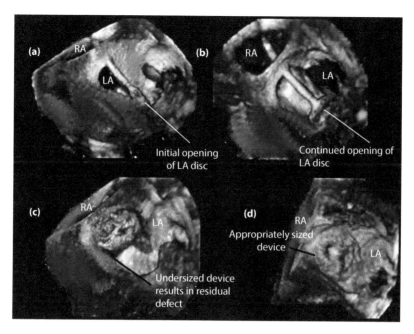

Figure 4.5 Intraprocedural RT3D TEE provides superior visualization of wires, catheters and devices and their relationship to neighbouring structures in a format that is generally better comprehended by the interventional cardiologist than 2D echocardiography. An ostium secundum ASD has been closed with an Amplatzer device under RT3D TEE guidance. All views are shown from the LA perspective. The LA disc of the device opening in the LA (a). View showing continued opening of the device (b). An undersized device with a residual defect (c). A larger closure device was used instead (d). (Adapted from ASE guidelines for echocardiographic assessment of ASD and PFO, August 2015.)

Intracardiac echocardiography has been used extensively to guide percutaneous ASD/PFO closure procedures and is the imaging modality of choice in many centres in the cardiac catheterization laboratory. The advantages of ICE include an image quality that is similar but not identical to that of TEE, facilitating a comprehensive assessment of the IAS, location and size of the defects, the adequacy of the rims and location of the pulmonary veins. It also retains an advantage compared with TEE in imaging the inferior and posterior portions of the IAS. Finally, the use of ICE eliminates the need for general anaesthesia and endotracheal intubation and can be performed with the patient under conscious sedation. An interventionalist can perform intracardiac echocardiography without the need for additional support personnel. However, the potential disadvantages of ICE include a limited far-field view, catheter instability, the expense of single-use ICE catheters, the need for additional training, the risk of provocation of atrial arrhythmias and increased technical difficulty for a single operator. Table 4.2 provides a summary of the advantages and disadvantages of TTE, TEE and ICE in percutaneous transcatheter guidance of PFO and ASD.

Transthoracic echocardiography protocol for imaging the interatrial septum[3]

The atrial septum can be evaluated fully using TTE. Multiple views should be used to evaluate the size, shape and location of an atrial communication and the relationship of the defect to its surrounding structures. In particular, special attention must be paid to determine the relationship of the defect to the venae cavae, pulmonary veins, mitral and tricuspid valves and coronary sinus. Assessment of the amount of the surrounding rims of tissue present is crucial. A deficiency of rim tissue between the defect and pulmonary veins, AV valve or IVC will preclude transcatheter closure, and a deficiency of aortic rim can increase the risk of device erosion in certain circumstances.

Table 4.2 Advantages and disadvantages of TTE, TEE and ICE in percutaneous transcatheter guidance of PFO and ASD

Modality	Advantages	Disadvantages
TTE	• Readily available • Low cost • Unlimited multiple planes to evaluate IAS • Non-invasive • Does not require any additional sedation • Excellent image quality in paediatric patients	• Image qualities in larger patients could be optimal • Requires technologist or echocardiographer to perform study during closure • Lower rim of IAS not well seen after device placement owing to shadowing in virtually all views
TEE	• Improved image quality over TTE • 3D technique adds incremental value over 2D technique in evaluating ASD size, shape, location • Provides en face imaging that might be more intuitively understood to non-imagers	• Requires additional sedation or anaesthesia to perform • Risks include aspiration and esophageal trauma • Could require endotracheal intubation if prolonged procedure • Requires additional echocardiographic operator to perform • Patient discomfort
ICE	• Comparable image quality to TEE • Can be performed with patient under conscious sedation • Reduces procedure and fluoroscopy times • Superior to TEE for evaluating inferior aspects of IAS • Interventionalist autonomy (without additional support)	• Invasive risks of 8F–10F venous access and catheter, including vascular risk and arrhythmia • Role of 3D technique to be defined • Cost of single-use ICE catheters • Limited far-field views with some systems • Need for additional training of ICE operator

Additional views of other structures, such as the ventricles and great arteries, are necessary to assess for secondary findings related to the hemodynamic consequences of an ASD such as RA, right ventricular (RV) and pulmonary artery (PA) dilation. In the paediatric population, the subxiphoid window typically allows the best visualization of the atrial septum and its related structures. In adolescence and adulthood, the subxiphoid window is often inadequate because of the distance from the probe to the atrial septum. Thus, other views such as the parasternal windows should be used to assess the atrial septum. In some cases, a full assessment of the atrial septum might not be possible with transthoracic echocardiogram, thus, transesophageal echo could be required.

SUBXIPHOID FRONTAL (FOUR-CHAMBER) TTE VIEW

The subxiphoid four-chamber view allows imaging of the atrial septum along its anterior–posterior axis from the SVC to the AV valves. This is the preferred view for imaging the atrial septum, because the atrial septum runs near perpendicularly to the ultrasound beam, providing the highest axial resolution and permitting measurement of the defect diameter along its long axis. Because the septum is thin (especially in its midportion), placing the septum perpendicular to the ultrasound beam helps distinguish a true defect from dropout resulting from an artefact. Aneurysms of the atrial septum primum composed of tissue attached to the edges of the ASD are also well visualized from the subcostal frontal view. ASAs could be fenestrated (Figure 4.6) but also can be intact with no resultant atrial level shunt. Colour Doppler interrogation and contrast studies should be used to detect shunting. The surrounding rim from the defect to the right pulmonary veins can be measured in this view. Sinus venosus defects are difficult to visualize because the vena cava is not viewed longitudinally in this view.

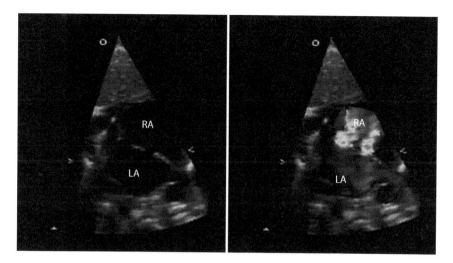

Figure 4.6 Subxiphoid TTE demonstrating multi fenestrated IAS without and with colour Doppler flow from left to right in a paediatric patient. (Adapted from ASE guidelines for echocardiographic assessment of ASD and PFO, August 2015.)

SUBXIPHOID SAGITTAL TTE VIEW

The subxiphoid sagittal transthoracic view is acquired by turning the transducer 90 degrees clockwise from the frontal view. The view is ideal for imaging of the atrial septum along its superior–inferior axis in a plane orthogonal to the subxiphoid frontal four-chamber view. Sweeping the transducer from right to left in this axis allows determination of the orthogonal dimensions of the ASD (Figures 4.7 and 4.8). These dimensions can be compared with the dimensions measured in the subxiphoid frontal view to help determine the shape (circular or oval) of the defect. This view can

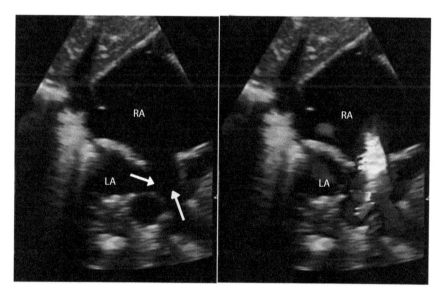

Figure 4.7 Transthoracic echocardiogram of a SVC type venosus ASD in subxiphoid sagittal view without and with colour in a paediatric patient. The yellow arrow represents the right superior pulmonary vein, and the white arrow the defect entering the atrium. (Adapted from ASE guidelines for echocardiographic assessment of ASD and PFO, August 2015.)

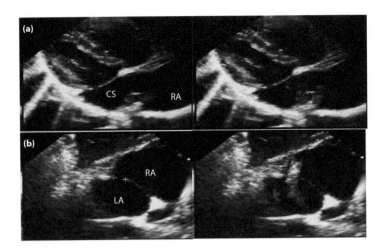

Figure 4.8 Two-dimensional TTE (left) and with colour Doppler (right) demonstrating unroofed coronary sinus interatrial communication in four-chamber view; dilated coronary sinus is seen (a). Two-dimensional TTE (left) and with colour Doppler (right) demonstrate unroofed coronary sinus with interatrial communication in subcostal left anterior oblique view (b). (Adapted from ASE guidelines for echocardiographic assessment of ASD and PFO, August 2015.)

be used to measure the rim from the defect to the SVC and IVC and is an excellent window to image a sinus venosus type defect (Figure 4.7 and 4.9).

LEFT ANTERIOR OBLIQUE TTE VIEW

The left anterior oblique TTE view is acquired by turning the transducer approximately 45° counter clockwise from the frontal (four-chamber) view.

This view allows imaging of the length of the atrial septum and is therefore ideal to identify ostium primum ASDs and for assessment of coronary sinus dilation (Figures 4.8b and 4.10b). In addition, it allows evaluation of the relation of the SVC to the defect. Furthermore, this view can be used to evaluate the entrance of the right-sided pulmonary veins into the heart.

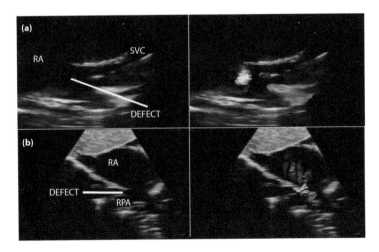

Figure 4.9 Representative example of 2D TTE (left) and with colour Doppler (right) of an SVC type sinus venosus ASD from the high right parasternal view (a). Representative example of 2D TTE (left) and with colour Doppler (right) of an SVC type sinus venosus ASD from the subcostal sagittal view; RPA, right pulmonary artery (b). (Adapted from ASE guidelines for echocardiographic assessment of ASD and PFO, August 2015.)

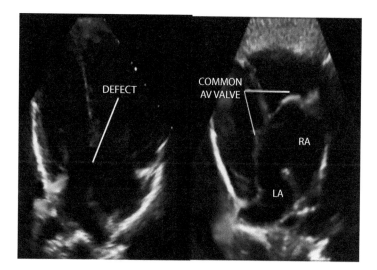

Figure 4.10 Primum ASD by 2D TTE in apical four-chamber view (a). Primum ASD by 2D TTE in subcostal left anterior oblique view; CAVV, common AV valve (b).

APICAL FOUR-CHAMBER TTE VIEW

In the apical four-chamber TTE view, the diagnosis and measurement of ASD should be avoided because the atrial septum is aligned parallel to the ultrasound beam. Thus, artefactual dropout is frequent in this view, which results in overestimation of the defect size. This view is better to assess the hemodynamic consequences of ASD, such as RA and RV dilation, and to estimate the RV pressure using the tricuspid valve regurgitant jet velocity. This view is also used to evaluate for right-to-left shunting with agitated saline[5] (Figure 4.11).

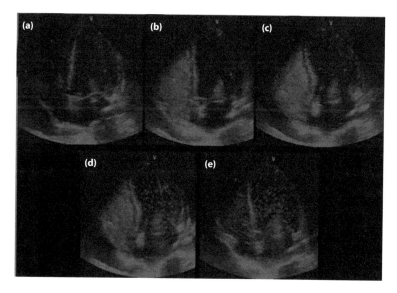

Figure 4.11 TTE of an apical four-chamber view during saline contrast injection. First images demonstrate prominent artefact over mitral valve (a). Opacification of the RA and RV (b). Delayed entry of contrast into the LA and LV, consistent with a pulmonary arteriovenous malformation; if the bubbles cross within the first three cardiac cycles, an intracardiac shunt is present (c). Subsequent cardiac cycles demonstrate continued opacification of the LA and LV consistent with intrapulmonary shunting (d and e). (Adapted from ASE guidelines for echocardiographic assessment of ASD and PFO, August 2015.)

MODIFIED APICAL FOUR-CHAMBER VIEW (HALF WAY BETWEEN APICAL FOUR-CHAMBER AND PARASTERNAL SHORT-AXIS TTE VIEW)

The modified apical four-chamber TTE view is obtained by sliding the transducer medially from the apical four-chamber view to the sternal border. This view highlights the atrial septum from an improved incidence angle to the sound beam (30°–45°). In the patients in whom the subcostal views are difficult to obtain, the modified apical four-chamber view is an alternative method for imaging the atrial septum in the direction of the axial resolution of the equipment.

PARASTERNAL SHORT-AXIS TTE VIEW

In the parasternal short-axis TTE view at the base of the heart, the atrial septum is visualized posterior to the aortic root running in an anterior–posterior orientation (Figure 4.12). This view is ideal to identify the aortic rim of the defect (Figures 4.13 and 4.14). It also highlights the posterior rim (or lack thereof) in sinus venosus and postero-inferior secundum defects. The size of the defect itself should not be measured in this view, because the beam orientation is parallel to the septum, and dropout resulting from artefact can occur.

HIGH RIGHT PARASTERNAL VIEW

The high right parasternal view is a modified para-sagittal view, performed with the patient in the right lateral decubitus position with the probe in the superior–inferior orientation. In this view, the atrial septum is aligned perpendicular to the beam and is ideal for diagnosing sinus venosus defects, particularly when the subxiphoid windows are inadequate (Figure 4.15).

TRANSESOPHAGEAL ECHOCARDIOGRAPHY IMAGING PROTOCOL FOR THE INTERATRIAL SEPTUM[2]

As with TTE, multiple and sequential TEE views should be used to completely and systematically evaluate the IAS, the size, shape and location of any atrial communication present and the relationship of the defect to its surrounding structures. Sequential interrogation and the digital capture of images starting from the standard views and then by

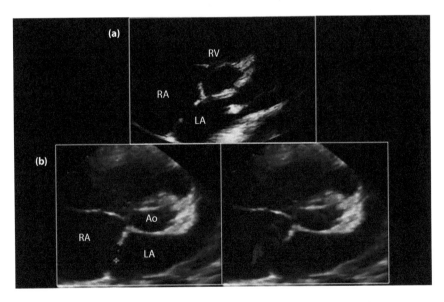

Figure 4.12 Two-dimensional TTE of ostium secundum ASD from parasternal short-axis view (a). Two-dimensional TTE (left) and with colour Doppler (right) of an ostium secundum ASD from the parasternal short-axis view with measurement of the diameter in the anterior–posterior orientation and left-to-right flow by colour Doppler. Ao, aortic root (b). (Adapted from ASE guidelines for echocardiographic assessment of ASD and PFO, August 2015.)

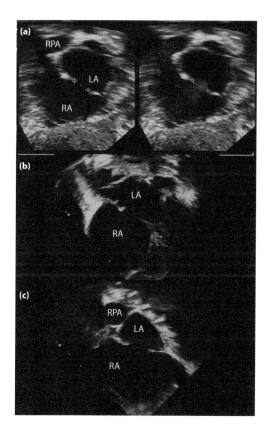

Figure 4.13 TTE of a secundum type ASD in the parasternal short-axis view without and with colour Doppler in a paediatric patient. (Adapted from ASE guidelines for echocardiographic assessment of ASD and PFO, August 2015.)

stepwise increases in the transducer angle in a series of 15° increments to pan or sweep the ultrasound beam through the areas of interest is recommended. Two-dimensional images should be optimized and colour Doppler mapping subsequently applied. The colour Doppler scale can be reduced slightly to approximately 35–40 cm/sec to capture low-velocity

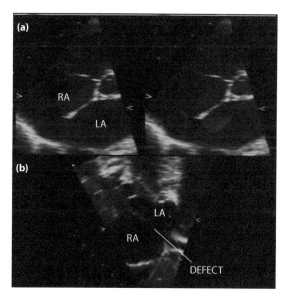

Figure 4.14 Examples of ostium secundum by 2D TTE (left) and with colour Doppler (right) in the subcostal left anterior oblique view (a and b). Measurement of the ASD diameter (left) and left-to-right colour Doppler flow (right). Sagittal subcostal view in a patient (c). (Adapted from ASE guidelines for echocardiographic assessment of ASD and PFO, August 2015.)

Figure 4.15 Inferior vena cava type sinus venosus ASD by 2D TTE (left) and with colour Doppler (right) in the parasternal short-axis view with left-to-right flow (a). IVC type sinus venosus ASD by 2D transthoracic echocardiography in the subcostal view (b). (Adapted from ASE guidelines for echocardiographic assessment of ASD and PFO, August 2015.)

Table 4.3 Key imaging views for evaluation of the interatrial septum and surrounding structures

View	Septal anatomy	Procedural assessment
Subxiphoid long-axis or left anterior oblique	Atrial septal right pulmonary vein rim, atrial septal defect diameter and atrial septal length	Position of device with regard to right pulmonary veins and assessment for residual leak
Subxiphoid short-axis (sagittal)	SVC and IVC rim and atrial septal defect diameter	Position of device with regard to SVC and IVC and assessment for residual leak
Apical four-chamber view	Rim of defect to AV valves, assessment of RV dilation. RV pressure estimate from tricuspid regurgitation jet velocity	Position of device with regard to AV valves
Parasternal short-axis	Position of device with regard to AV valves	Device relationship to aortic valve, assessment for impingement on aorta or straddle and relationship of device to posterior wall

flow across a small fenestration, PFO or smaller ASD. Pulsed and continuous-wave Doppler should then be used to measure the velocity, direction and timing of flow in the representative views. TTE for the evaluation of the IAS and surrounding structures is summarized in Table 4.3.

Capturing 3D volumes with and without colour Doppler of the IAS allows for even greater data acquisition without the need for sequential multiplane. When an ASD or PFO is present, attention must be given to determining the relationship of the defect to the venae cava, pulmonary veins, mitral and tricuspid valves and coronary sinus. An assessment of the amount of the surrounding

rims of tissue is critical for evaluation of patient candidacy for percutaneous transcatheter closure. A deficient rim is defined as less than 5 mm in multiple sequential views, and this should be evaluated in at least three sequential related multiplane views in 15° increments. As with TTE, additional views of the other cardiac structures are necessary to assess for secondary findings related to the hemodynamic consequences of an ASD such as right heart and pulmonary arterial dilation. When using TEE, five base views are used to assess the IAS and surrounding structures, summarized in Table 4.4. These key views include the upper esophageal short-axis view, midesophageal aortic

Table 4.4 Views for assessment of ASD by TEE

View	Atrial septal anatomy	Procedural assessment	Suggested multiplane angles	Esophageal position
Basal transverse	SVC, superior aortic, RUPV	Device relationship in atrial roof	0°, 15°, 30°, 45°	Mid to upper oesophagus
Four-chamber	Posterior and AV rims, maximal ASD diameter	Device relationship to AV valves	0°, 15°, 30°	Midesophagus
Short-axis	Posterior and aortic rims, maximal ASD diameter	Device relationship to AoV and posterior atrial wall	30°, 45°, 60°, 75°	Mid to upper oesophagus
Bicaval	IVC and SVC rims, maximal ASD diameter	Device relationship to RA roof or dome.	90°,120°	Midesophagus and deep transgastric.
Long-axis	Dome or roof of left atrium.	Device relationship to LA roof/dome	120°, 135°, 150°	Mid to upper oesophagus

valve (AoV) short-axis view, midesophageal four-chamber view, midesophageal bicaval view and midesophageal long-axis view.

UPPER ESOPHAGEAL SHORT-AXIS VIEW

The upper esophageal short-axis view is obtained from the upper oesophagus starting at multiplane angles of 0°, with stepwise sweeping and recording at 15°, 30° and 45°. This view facilitates imaging of the superior aspects of the atrial septum, including the septum secundum, the roofs of the RA and LA and the surrounding great vessels (SVC and ascending aorta). Entry of the right pulmonary veins can be demonstrated by insertion into the midesophagus and by clockwise rotation of the probe in these views (Figure 4.16). Anomalous pulmonary venous drainage and SVC type of sinus venosus defect are noted in the given view.

MIDESOPHAGEAL AORTIC VALVE SHORT-AXIS VIEW

The midesophageal aortic valve short-axis view is obtained from the midesophagus starting with a multiplane angle of approximately 30° and stepwise sweeping

through and recording additional views at 45°, 60° and 75°. This progression of transducer angles allows transitional interrogation of the IAS from the AoV short-axis view to the modified bicaval tricuspid valve view. The AoV short-axis view is typically obtained to present short-axis views of the AoV and its surrounding septum. This view facilitates imaging of the anterior and posterior planes of the atrial septum (and aortic and posterior rims if an ASD is present), the antero-posterior diameter of the ASD and the overlap of septum primum and septum secundum when a PFO is present (Figures 4.17 and 4.18) (Adapted from ASE guidelines for echocardiographic assessment of ASD and PFO, August 2015)

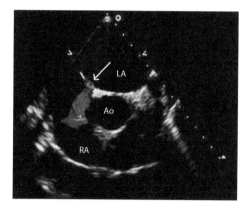

Figure 4.17 TEE of small ostium secundum ASD (yellow arrow) at the midesophageal aortic valve short-axis view from the midesophagus. Ao, ascending aorta. (Adapted from ASE guidelines for echocardiographic assessment of ASD and PFO, August 2015.)

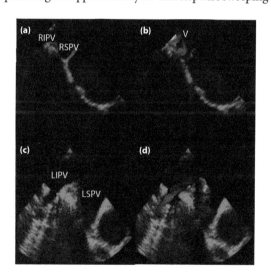

Figure 4.16 TEE demonstrating from the upper esophageal short-axis view demonstrating the right pulmonary veins at 0° without (a) and with colour Doppler (b) and at 60° without (c) and with colour Doppler (d). (Adapted from ASE guidelines for echocardiographic assessment of ASD and PFO, August 2015.)

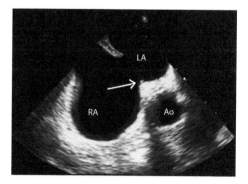

Figure 4.18 TEE of large ostium secundum ASD from midesophageal AoV short-axis view. Short-axis view of ostium secundum ASD. Note aortic rim (arrow). AV, aortic valve/aorta. (Adapted from ASE guidelines for echocardiographic assessment of ASD and PFO, August 2015.)

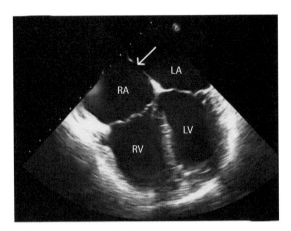

Figure 4.19 TEE of large ostium secundum ASD from midesophageal four-chamber view; note ASD (white arrow). (Adapted from ASE guidelines for echocardiographic assessment of ASD and PFO, August 2015.)

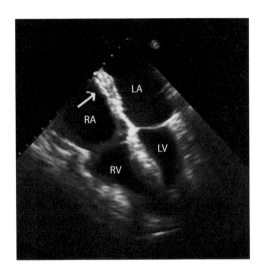

Figure 4.20 TEE of closure device in ostium secundum ASD from midesophageal four-chamber view; note relationship between AV valves; note ASD closure device (yellow arrow). (Adapted from ASE guidelines for echocardiographic assessment of ASD and PFO, August 2015.)

Midesophageal four-chamber view

The midesophageal four-chamber view is obtained from the midesophagus, beginning with a multiplane angles of 0° and stepwise increases of the multiplane angle to 15° and 30°. This view is used to evaluate the AV septum (deficient in primum ASD) and the relationship of any ASD to the AV valves (Figure 4.19). Larger devices used to close secundum ASD can interfere or impinge on AV valve function, and this must be carefully evaluated before device deployment (Figure 4.20).

The midesophageal bicaval view used to image the inferior and superior planes of the atrial septum and the surrounding structures, the SVC and right pulmonary veins (Figures 4.21, 4.22, and 4.23) is obtained at the midesophagus level with multiplane angles from 90°, 105° and 120°. This view is important for evaluating sinus venosus defects of the SVC type and also for assessing for anomalous pulmonary vein. This view is also important in evaluating the roof or dome of the

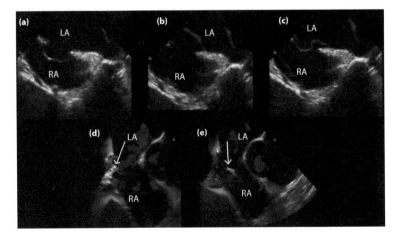

Figure 4.21 Two-dimensional TEE (bicaval view) of IAS with ASA demonstrating excessive mobility of the fossa ovalis (a–c) and associated multiple fenestrations (d–e) (yellow arrows). (Adapted from ASE guidelines for echocardiographic assessment of ASD and PFO, August 2015.)

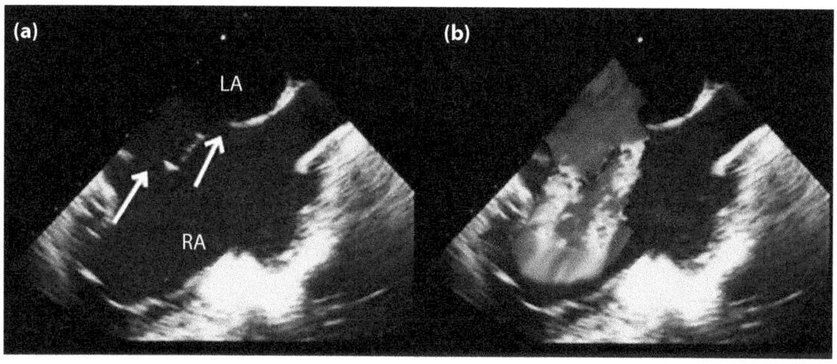

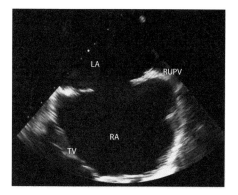

Figure 4.22 Bicaval view demonstrating two discrete ASDs **(a)**. Bicaval view with color Doppler demonstrating two discrete left-to-right shunts **(b)**. (Adapted from ASE guidelines for echocardiographic assessment of ASD and PFO, August 2015.)

Figure 4.23 TEE of large ostium secundum ASD from midesophageal modified bicaval view (includes the tricuspid valve). (Adapted from ASE guidelines for echocardiographic assessment of ASD and PFO, August 2015.)

RA, which must be visualized before release of ASD closure devices.

Midesophageal long-axis view

The midesophageal long-axis view is obtained from the midesophagus with multiplane angles of 120°, 135° and 150° to evaluate the roof or dome of the LA when a percutaneous device is placed. (See the section 'Role of Echocardiography in Percutaneous Transcatheter Device Closure'.) Rotation past the LA appendage demonstrates the entry of the left pulmonary veins into the LA. (Figure 4.24)

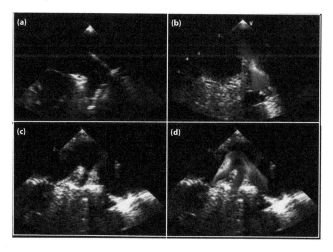

Figure 4.24 Midesophageal views **(a)** without and **(b)** with colour Doppler obtained at 60° (mitral commissural view) with the probe then rotated to the left to reveal the left pulmonary veins. Midesophageal long-axis views with the probe rotated towards the left pulmonary veins at 120° **(c)** without and **(d)** with colour flow Doppler. (Adapted from ASE guidelines for echocardiographic assessment of ASD and PFO, August 2015.)

3D TEE acquisition protocol for PFO and ASD

Three-dimensional transesophageal images of the IAS should be acquired from multiple views and multiple 3D imaging modes for analysis.[9] A comprehensive 3D echocardiography examination usually starts with a real-time or narrow-angled acquisition from the standard imaging views. To obtain images with higher temporal and spatial resolution, electrocardiographically gated, 3D wide-angled acquisitions are then performed. When evaluating the IAS using TEE, narrow-angled, zoomed and wide-angled acquisition of 3D data from several key views is recommended.

Midesophageal short-axis view—This view is acquired from the midesophagus starting at a multiplane angle of 0°. The probe is rotated towards the IAS. This view is particularly suited to narrow- and wide-angled acquisitions.

Basal short-axis view—This view is acquired from the midesophagus starting at 30° to 60° multiplane angles. It is particularly suited for narrow- and wide-angled acquisitions. This view also facilitates zoom mode imaging during procedure guidance. Processing the 3D images from this view facilitates the demonstration of an ASD en face and demonstrates the relationship to the surrounding structures (e.g., the aorta and aortic rim) (Figures 4.25 and 4.26a and 4.26b). Wide-angled acquisition from this view should be acquired with and without colour Doppler flow mapping for precise offline measurements of ASD size, shape, dynamic change and relationship to surrounding structures.

Bicaval view—This view is acquired from the midesophageal level with the transducer starting at the 90° to 120° in multiplane orientation. This view can also be captured by each of the 3D imaging modalities. The depth of pyramidal data sets should be adjusted to include only the left and right sides of the atrial septum in this view. This specific setting will allow the entire septum to be acquired in a 3D format without incorporating the surrounding structures. With a perpendicular up–down angulation of the data set, the left-sided aspect of the septum can be shown in an en face

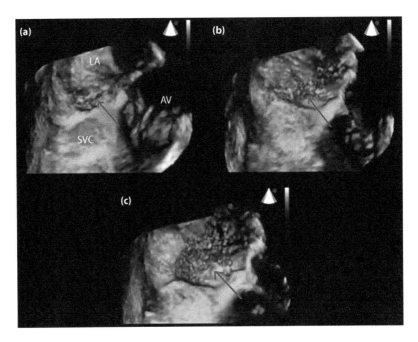

Figure 4.25 Real-time 3D TEE images from the midesophageal short-axis views of a PFO during a saline contrast study. The PFO exit into the LA is apparent (blue arrow). This is performed to help localize the site of bubble entry into the LA and not to quantify the size of the shunt. Progressive saline contrast microbubbles crossing through the PFO into the LA (a–c). Blue arrow specifies PFO tunnel. (Adapted from ASE guidelines for echocardiographic assessment of ASD and PFO, August 2015.)

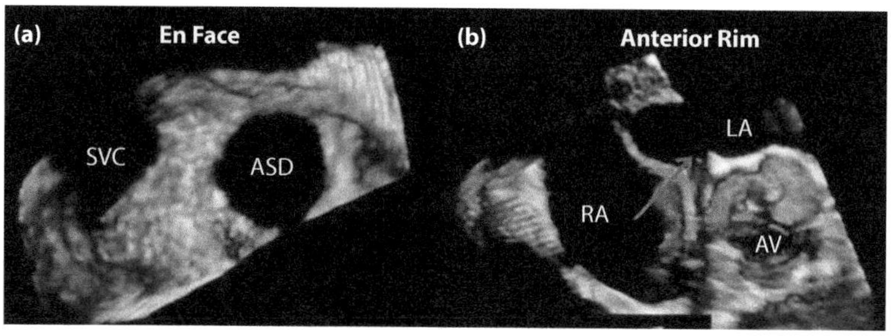

(a) En Face	(b) Anterior Rim

SVC ASD

LA
RA
AV

Figure 4.26 Real-time 3D TEE images of an ostium secundum ASD from the RA perspective demonstrating an ASD en face from the midesophageal short-axis view (a) and RA perspective demonstrating the aortic rim (arrow) from the midesophageal short-axis view (b). (Adapted from ASE guidelines for echocardiographic assessment of ASD and PFO, August 2015.)

view (Figure 4.27). Once the left side of the atrial septum has been acquired, a 180° counter clockwise rotation will show the right side of the atrial septum

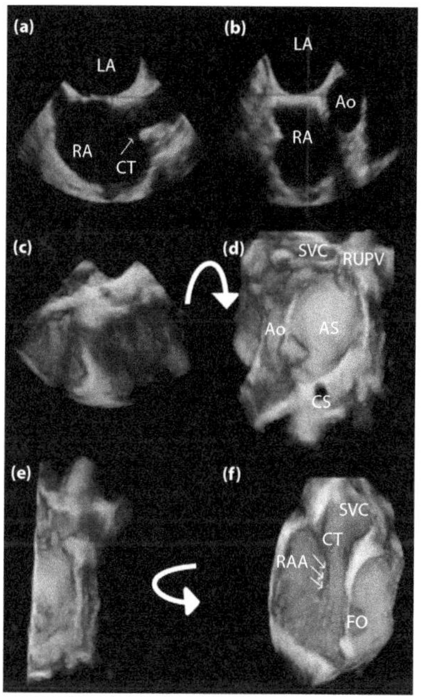

Figure 4.27 Still image depicting the two perpendicular 2D TEE planes (a and b) used to acquire a zoomed 3DE data set of the IAS (c). The left side of the atrial septum is shown in the en face perspective visualized after a 90° up–down rotation (curved arrow) of the data set (d). Image (d) can be cropped to remove the left half of the atrial septum (e) and when rotated 90° counter clockwise (curved arrow) (f), the entire course of the crista terminalis from the SVC towards the IVC (arrows) can be visualized. (Adapted from ASE guidelines for echocardiographic assessment of ASD and PFO, August 2015.)

and the fossa ovalis as a depression on the septum (Figure 4.28). Sometimes the use of fine cropping using the arbitrary crop plane will be necessary to remove the surrounding atrial structures that can obscure the septum. Again, setting at medium level is usually required to avoid the disappearance of the fossa ovalis and creating a false impression of an ASD. This view is also used to measure the size and shape of the ASD in systole and diastole.

Sagittal bicaval view—This can be obtained from the deep transgastric position with a transducer orientation of 100° to 120°. The recommendations for the settings and processing of this view are identical to that of the midesophageal bicaval view.

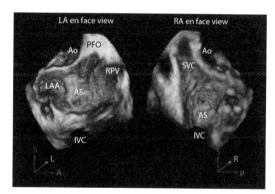

Figure 4.28 The interatrial septum when viewed from the LA (left). The atrial septum should be oriented with the right upper pulmonic vein at the 1 o'clock position. When displayed as viewed from the right atrium (right), the SVC should be located at the 11 o'clock position. A, anterior; AS, atrial septum, Ao, aorta; L, left; LAA, left atrial appendage; P, posterior; R, right; S, superior. (Adapted from ASE guidelines for echocardiographic assessment of ASD and PFO, August 2015.)

Four-chamber view—This view is acquired from the midesophageal level starting at 0° to 20° transducer orientations.

3D TTE ACQUISITION PROTOCOL FOR PFO AND ASD

Transthoracic 3D images of the IAS can be obtained from the narrow-angle apical four-chamber, narrow-angle parasternal long-axis colour and apical four-chamber zoom views. However, image resolution can limit its utility in larger paediatric and adult patients.

3D DISPLAY

When the IAS is viewed from the LA (left), the atrial septum should be oriented with the right upper pulmonary vein at the 1 o'clock position. When displayed as viewed from the RA (right), the SVC should be located at the 11 o'clock position (Figures 4.27 and 4.28).

Images should be acquired from these transducer positions as an initial starting point using all three 3D echocardiographic modes, including narrow-angled, zoomed and wide-angled gated 3D acquisition modes.

In still images that are carefully acquired and cropped, it will not always be apparent which 3D echocardiographic mode was used. In video images, the 3D zoomed acquisition mode will be noticeable by its slow volume rate and smooth images, and the 3D wide-angled gated acquisition mode will be noticeable by stitch artefacts, if present.

The qualitative anatomic parameters delineated from the 3D data set should include the type of ASD (e.g., secundum, primum, sinus venosus, coronary sinus or common atrium), location within the atrial septum, shape and orientation. The ASD shape can be defined as oval, round, triangular or, at times, shaped somewhat like an egg/pear or slightly irregular. The ASD orientation is usually defined according to the long-axis orientation of the defect as vertical, horizontal, oblique with an anterior tilt or oblique with a posterior tilt. Defects in which the lengths of the long-axis and short-axis dimensions are within 1 mm should be designated as round.

Quantitative analysis of ASD using 3D echocardiography should include the maximum length, width and area measured at atrial end-diastole (Figure 4.29). The ASD dimensions should also

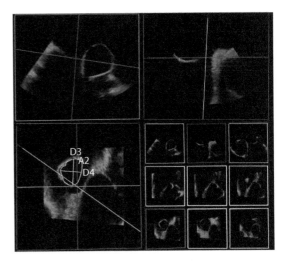

Figure 4.29 Once 3D volumes are acquired, post-processing using commercially available 3D software packages will align the plane of the IAS with multiple 3D plane slices. This approach facilitates an assessment of the shape of an ASD and allows for measurement of en face diameters and area in multiple orthogonal views, without the potential for bias due to malalignment of the ultrasound planes. (Adapted from ASE guidelines for echocardiographic assessment of ASD and PFO, August 2015.)

be measured at atrial end-systole to determine the change in the dimensions during the cardiac cycle (dynamic ASD). The ASD dimensions are measured in en face views from either the RA or LA perspective using dedicated quantitative software. The parameters calculated can include the percentage of change in ASD length, width and area from atrial end-diastole to atrial end-systole. Atrial end-diastole is defined as the frame with the largest ASD dimension and atrial end-systole as the frame with the smallest ASD dimension. The number of defects in the atrial septum should be quantified if multiple.

Intracardiac echocardiographic imaging protocol for IAS

A comprehensive assessment of the atrial septum, septal defects and surrounding tissue rims can be performed with radial or phased array ICE. The key ICE views used in the evaluation of the IAS as described are listed in Table 4.5.

Table 4.5 Intracardiac echocardiographic views for assessment of IAS

ICE view	Position of ICE catheter	Anterior–posterior flexion	Right–left flexion	Visualized structures
Home view	Mid-right atrium	Neutral	Neutral	RA, TV, RV, PV, RVOT, lower IAS
Septal view	Mid-right atrium	Posterior deflection	Rightward	Inferior and superior IAS, septum primum, septum secundum, relationship to MV
Septal long-axis or bicaval	Upper right atrium	Posterior deflection	Rightward	IAS, septum primum, septum secundum, SVC
Septal short-axis	Mid-right atrium, turn towards tricuspid valve	Posterior deflection	Leftward	Aortic Valve, IAS, posterior–anterior plane of ASD, posterior and AV rims

The currently available intracardiac echocardiography systems do not have electronic beam steering or multiplane transducer angle capabilities. Instead, they offer a radial rotational or phased area imaging plane that is manipulated by insertion and withdrawal of the catheter, axial rotation and, in the case of the phased array systems, by manipulating the steering controls with adjustable tension such that the catheter can be held in a flexed position in up to four directions (anterior, posterior, left and right). Insertion and withdrawal of the phased array ICE probe will result in imaging more superiorly and inferiorly, and axial rotation allows for sweeping the image through multiple planes. Three-dimensional ICE has recently become commercially available. Limited data exist regarding the role of 3D ICE in percutaneous transcatheter procedures at present. The use of 3D ICE offers the potential to provide greater anatomic information during structural interventions but requires additional investigation to fully define its role.[10]

The phased array ICE probe is initially positioned in the mid-RA in a neutral catheter position to visualize the tricuspid valve in the long axis. This is referred to as the 'home view' (Figure 4.30a). In this view, the RA, tricuspid valve, RV, RVOT, pulmonary valve, proximal main pulmonary artery, a portion of the AoV and any ASD that is present with the adjacent septum in the partial short-axis view can be identified. This view also visualizes the lower portion of the atrioventricular (AV) septal rim.

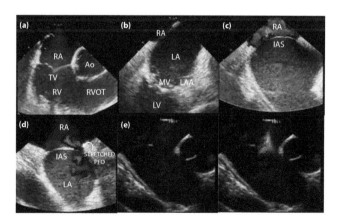

Figure 4.30 Intracardiac echocardiographic evaluation of the IAS. Home view (a). Septal long-axis view (b). Bicaval view (c). Septal short-axis view of PFO (d). Septal short-axis view of ostium secundum ASD (e). The white arrow specifies the direction of PFO flow through stretched PFO. IAS, interatrial septum; LAA, left atrial appendage; RA, right atrium; RVOT, right ventricular outflow tract; TV, tricuspid valve. (Adapted from ASE guidelines for echocardiographic assessment of ASD and PFO, August 2015.)

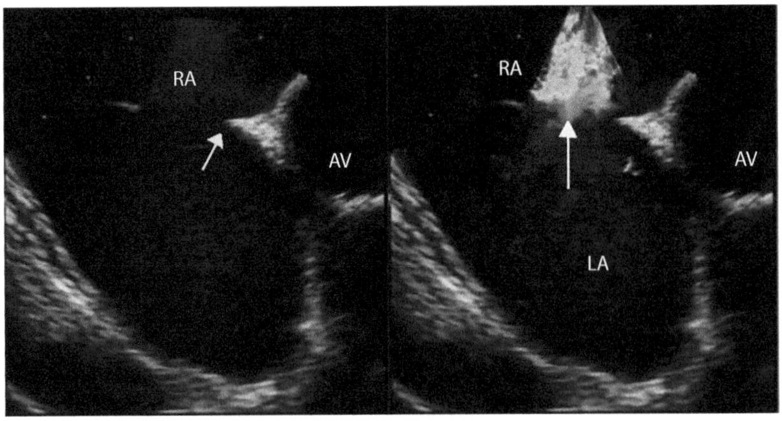

Figure 4.31 Intracardiac echocardiogram of an ostium secundum ASD with left-to-right flow with and without colour Doppler mapping. The white arrow specifies the direction of ASD flow; yellow arrow, the aortic rim. AV, aortic valve. (Adapted from ASE guidelines for echocardiographic assessment of ASD and PFO, August 2015.)

From this position, applying posterior deflection of the posterior–anterior knob and applying slight rightward rotation of the right–left knob will obtain the septal long-axis view (Figure 4.30b). Advancing the catheter cephalad will produce a bicaval view from which the superior and inferior rims of an ASD and the defect diameter and configuration can be measured. (Figure 4.30c).

Rotation of the entire catheter handle clockwise until the intracardiac transducer is near the tricuspid valve, followed by slight leftward rotation of the right–left knob until the AoV appears, creates a septal short-axis view similar to the TEE short-axis plane, with the difference being that the near field in the present view is the RA compared with TEE showing the LA (Figure 4.30d and 4.30e). From this view, the diameter of the defect and the anterior (aortic) and posterior rims can be measured (Figure 4.31).

There is, however, no true four-chamber view, because the ICE catheter sits in the RA.

ASSESSMENT OF SHUNTING

Techniques, characterization, standards and visualization of shunting: TTE and TEE

Shunting, and the hemodynamic significance of shunting, across an ASD or PFO is evaluated through a combination of structural imaging, colour flow Doppler mapping and spectral Doppler

interrogation. Associated findings, including diastolic flattening of the ventricular septum and dilatation of the RA, RV and/or PA, are all potential signs of significant left-to-right shunting. The severity of dilatation is related to the relative compliance of these structures, as well as to the size of the ASD.

The direction of shunting though an ASD is usually left to right and is visualized using colour flow Doppler. ASD shunt flow can be right to left or bidirectional in the setting of significant pulmonary hypertension or significant impairment of RV compliance.[11] Pulse-wave spectral Doppler can be used for the detection of bidirectional shunting, in addition to colour Doppler. The colour scale settings should be adjusted to optimize for the expected low velocity of shunting (i.e., 25–40 cm/sec). Occasionally, higher velocity left-to-right shunting will be present owing to LA hypertension from mitral stenosis, impaired left ventricular (LV) compliance or LV outflow obstruction. In patients with ASD, measurement of the maximal dimension (width) using colour Doppler has been correlated with the maximal dimension of the defect orifice when measured surgically. For example, in a small series of patients undergoing surgery, the TTE- and TEE-measured ASD colour flow Doppler jet width measurements demonstrated correlation with the anatomic maximal dimension observed at surgery. Both TTE and TEE colour flow Doppler echocardiography of the maximal jet width correlates with direct surgical measurement of the defect and, therefore, might provide an estimation of the ASD diameter. Significant pitfalls exist when solely using the diameters measured by colour Doppler to evaluate the size of an ASD; therefore, 2D or 3D measurements without colour should be relied on. The variability in colour quality between machine vendors and the variable colour settings can result in excessive colour bleed over the atrial septal tissue, resulting in an overestimation of the true defect size.

Shunt flow can be estimated by pulsed Doppler quantification of the pulmonary (Qp) to systemic (Qs) blood flow ratio. This is typically performed by pulse-wave Doppler using TTE by interrogation of the RV and LV outflow tracts. The method involves measurement of the systolic velocity time integrals (VTIs) of the RV and LV outflow and the maximal systolic diameters of the pulmonary and LV outflow regions. The diameters are then used for calculation of the corresponding outflow tract areas, assuming the outflow region to be circular. The mathematical estimation of the area of the RV and LV outflow tract multiplied by the corresponding VTI estimates the stroke volume for the right and left ventricle, respectively. The Qp/Qs ratio estimation is then the ratio of the pulmonary to systemic stroke volumes (RV stroke volume/LV stroke volume). This method has been validated and compared with oximetric methods in a small number of patients with secundum ASD, including those with pulmonary hypertension, mitral and tricuspid regurgitation, ventricular septal defect and Eisenmenger complex. Semilunar valve regurgitation modifies the stroke volume in proportion to the degree of regurgitation and can limit the estimation of shunt flow when a significant degree of regurgitation is present. A similar method has been used with inflow velocity and AV valve annular dimensions in diastole and also correlated with oximetric methods. Colour flow Doppler can also detect shunting across a PFO; however, the shunting is often intermittent and might not be readily detectable using colour flow Doppler. When a PFO is stretched by differences in the LA and RA pressure, a left-to-right colour Doppler shunt might be seen. First-generation contrast echocardiography with agitated saline combined with physiologic manoeuvres to provoke right-to-left shunting increases the sensitivity of PFO detection.[12] The microbubbles generated with agitation are too large to pass through normal pulmonary vasculature

and are easily detected by echocardiographic imaging because of their increased echogenicity[13] (Figure 4.11). The provocative manoeuvres used to transiently increase RA pressure include the Valsalva manoeuvre and cough. TTE with first-generation contrast can be used to detect PFOs with reasonable sensitivity and specificity; however, TEE is considered the reference standard for detection of a PFO. Whether using TTE or TEE, the accuracy of the test will be improved by the use of a standardized protocol that includes multiple injections of agitated saline with provocative manoeuvres to transiently increase the RA pressure. The appearance of microbubbles in the LA within 3–6 cardiac beats after opacification of the RA is considered positive for the presence of an intracardiac shunt such as a PFO (Figure 4.11). Ideally, bubbles will be visualized crossing the atrial septum through the PFO. Physiologic manoeuvres to transiently increase RA pressure are typically required to promote right-to-left shunting of microbubbles to identify a PFO when no shunting is present without provocation. The Valsalva manoeuvre using held expiration and release is one common manoeuvre performed. The Valsalva strain must be held long enough for microbubbles to fill the RA. The effectiveness of the Valsalva manoeuvre can be assessed echocardiographically by the presence of a leftward shift of the atrial septum with release of Valsalva, indicating the achievement of RA pressure greater than LA pressure. The appearance of microbubbles in the LA after 3–6 cardiac beats specifies intrapulmonary shunting, such as an arteriovenous malformation. Intrapulmonary shunting is confirmed when the bubbles are visualized entering the LA from the pulmonary veins and not visualized crossing the atrial septum. Other reasons for a false-positive bubble study for PFO are sinus venosus septal defect or other unidentified ASD or pseudo-contrast caused by the strain phase of Valsalva with transient stagnation of blood in the pulmonary veins. Bubble studies can result in false-negative findings because of inadequate opacification of the RA, an inadequate Valsalva manoeuvre, the presence of a Eustachian valve directing venous return from the IVC to the atrial septum (preventing microbubbles entering from the SVC to cross the atrial septum), an inability to increase the RA pressure above the LA pressure such as in the presence of LV diastolic dysfunction and poor image quality. In patients with poor image quality, the use of second-harmonic imaging can improve the identification and detection of microbubbles. Digital compression algorithms can decrease the sensitivity for detection of small intracardiac shunts, and some laboratories have continued to record contrast studies on analogue videocassette to maximize the sensitivity for the detection of small shunts.

Specific routes of saline contrast administration can be used in specific clinical scenarios for bubble studies. For example, a left antecubital vein saline contrast injection can be used to diagnose a persistent left SVC draining into the coronary sinus. Leg vein saline contrast administration can be used in the adult patient who has undergone ASD closure but has persistent cyanosis after the procedure because an inferior sinus venosus ASD might have been incompletely closed, with persistence of IVC flow into the LA. A leg vein injection also can rarely be used to overcome a very large Chiari or Eustachian network that might impede the bubbles entering the RA from the SVC.

Sedated patients may not be able to perform an adequate Valsalva manoeuvre. In that circumstance, pressure on the abdomen can be applied to transiently increase the RA pressure. If the patient is under general anaesthesia, the Valsalva manoeuvre can be mimicked by held inspiration and then release. Reports have included attempted quantification of right-to-left shunting based on the number of microbubbles appearing in the left heart on an echocardiographic still frame; however, this number is dependent on the amount of microbubbles injected and the adequacy of the Valsalva manoeuvre.

Transcranial Doppler detection/ grading of shunting

Transcranial Doppler is an alternative imaging method for the detection of a PFO. This method uses power M-mode Doppler interrogation of the basal cerebral arteries to detect microbubbles that have crossed right to left into the systemic circulation.[14] Specialized equipment is used to focus the ultrasound system and display the results. As with contrast-enhanced TTE and TEE, TCD studies are performed with normal respiration and with the Valsalva manoeuvre to maximize the sensitivity and specificity of the test.[15] The results are reported referenced to a six-level Spencer logarithmic scale,

and higher grades have been associated with larger right-to-left shunts. The advantages of TCD over TEE and TTE include increased patient comfort (compared with TEE), semiquantitative assessment of shunt size and the ability to identify extracardiac and intracardiac shunting.[14] The identification of extracardiac shunts is also a limitation of TCD, because no anatomic information is provided regarding the location of the shunt or associated abnormalities. Hence, TCD and contrast echocardiography can be complementary techniques for the evaluation of right-to-left shunting. Some laboratories prefer to combine modalities and perform simultaneous contrast-enhanced TTE or TEE with TCD.[16] The detection and grading of shunting by any technique is complicated by physiologic variations in the presence and/or timing of the shunting. Respiratory phasic changes in RA pressure can result in delayed right-to-left shunting and misclassification of interatrial flow as an intrapulmonary shunt. Elevated LA pressure from LV failure, mitral stenosis or mitral regurgitation can prevent right-to-left shunting, because higher RA pressure is required to overcome the elevated LA pressure. In a study comparing patients with versus without left heart disease, the detection of PFO was 5% in the patients with left heart disease and 29% in those without left heart disease, similar to that in the general population.

Impact of shunting on the right ventricle

The hemodynamic effects of ASD are primarily related to the direction and magnitude of shunting, which is determined by the size of the defect, the relative compliance of the RVs and LVs and the relative systemic and pulmonary vascular resistances. In most patients, the greater compliance of the RV compared with the LV, and the lower resistance of the pulmonary compared with the systemic circulation, results in a net left-to-right shunt. The most pronounced echocardiographic finding associated with this left-to-right shunt is dilatation of the RV. Right ventricle dimensions are best measured from an RV–focused apical four-chamber view. Although care should be taken to obtain the image which demonstrates the maximum diameter of the RV without any foreshortening. This can be accomplished by ensuring that the crux and apex of the heart are both in the view. An RV diameter greater than 41 mm at the base and greater than 35 mm at the mid-level specifies right ventricle dilatation. Similarly, a longitudinal dimension greater than 83 mm specifies RV enlargement. The RV area has been shown to correlate with the cardiac magnetic resonance-derived RV volume and can serve as a semiquantitative surrogate for the identification of RV dilatation. The 3D echocardiographically derived RV volume is the most accurate echocardiographic method to estimate the RV volume compared with cardiac magnetic resonance. Compared with 2D techniques, 3D echocardiography results in better reproducibility and less under estimation of the RV volume. An RV end-diastolic volume indexed to the body surface area of 87 mL/m² or greater for men and 74 mL/m² or greater for women is considered increased. In the setting of significant RV dilatation, it can be difficult to enclose the entire RV in the 3D volume of interest for calculation of the volume.

The interventricular septal shape/ventricular configuration is another marker of RV size. As the RV dilates in the setting of volume overload, such as left-to-right shunting through an ASD, the interventricular septum becomes displaced towards the LV in diastole, resulting in a flattened appearance compared with the normal round appearance in the normal heart. In addition to the diastolic septal flattening associated with RV volume overload, systolic septal flattening can also be present in those patients with an ASD who have associated pulmonary hypertension. Visual assessment of the diastolic and systolic ventricular septal curvature, looking for a D-shaped pattern, should be used to help in the diagnosis of RV volume and/or pressure overload. Although a D-shaped ventricle formed by flattening of the septum is not diagnostic in RV overload. With its presence, additional emphasis should be placed on the confirmation, as well as the determination, of the aetiology and severity of right-sided pressure and/or volume overload. The severity of septal flattening increases with increasing RV dilatation and has been quantified with an eccentricity index derived from the perpendicular LV minor axis dimensions from the parasternal short-axis view. The ratio of the minor axis diameter parallel to the ventricular septum compared with the minor axis diameter that bisects the ventricular septum can be calculated at end-diastole. A ratio greater than one is associated with RV volume overload.

Pulmonary artery hypertension

The pulmonary vasculature normally accommodates the increased volume of flow secondary to ASD without a significant increase in PA pressure. With continued RV volume overload and increased PA flow over time, a small percentage of patients will develop pulmonary hypertension, with an even smaller percentage developing irreversible pulmonary vascular disease. This type of ASD is also associated with the frequency and rapidity of development of pulmonary hypertension, with the sinus venosus defect more frequently associated with pulmonary hypertension than secundum ASD and at younger ages. Evaluation for pulmonary hypertension is therefore an important part of the echocardiographic evaluation of an ASD before intervention. The systolic PA pressure is best estimated from the RV systolic pressure using the tricuspid regurgitation jet velocity (V) and the simplified Bernoulli equation: RV systolic pressure $= 4(V)^2 +$ estimated RA pressure. The normal peak RV systolic pressure should be less than 30–35 mm of Hg. The PA diastolic pressure can be similarly estimated from the pulmonary regurgitation end-diastolic velocity, and the mean PA pressure can be estimated from the peak PA velocity. Although accurate estimates of PA pressure can be calculated using non-invasive techniques, non-invasive estimation of the pulmonary vascular resistance is more problematic. However, it has been described using a ratio of peak tricuspid regurgitation velocity (in metres per second) compared with the RV outflow tract VTI (in centimetres).

RV function

In general, RV function (systolic or diastolic) is not adversely affected by the presence of an ASD; however, in some settings, RV function will be impaired, such as in the presence of significant pulmonary hypertension. When an evaluation of RV systolic function is required, the methods available include dP/dt, myocardial performance index, tricuspid annular plane systolic excursion, RV fractional area change, RV ejection fraction from 3D volumetric evaluation, Doppler tissue imaging (DTI) S' velocity, DTI isovolumic myocardial acceleration and deformation evaluation with RV strain and strain rate. For evaluation of RV diastolic function, the methods include transtricuspid

E and A wave velocities, E/A ratio, DTI E' and A' velocities, E/E' ratio, isovolumic relaxation time and deceleration time.

LV function

Age-related LV diastolic dysfunction can lead to increased left-to-right shunting across an ASD, with associated worsening of RV volume overload and late presentation of symptoms in older adults. These patients are at definite risk of developing acute heart failure with pulmonary oedema after closure of the ASD. This acute presentation is thought to be secondary to the combination of acute volume loading of the left heart in the setting of LV diastolic dysfunction that becomes unmasked with closure of the ASD. Pre-procedural echocardiographic evaluation of LV diastolic function with assessment of mitral inflow and annular velocities can identify some of these patients at risk of post-ASD closure heart failure and pulmonary congestion. However, LV diastolic dysfunction can be masked by the ASD and pressure equalization between the left heart and right heart. In those cases, invasive test occlusion of the ASD and measurement of the LA pressure can identify those patients at risk of developing pulmonary oedema. Pre-ASD closure treatment with diuretics and afterload reduction will help prevent post-ASD closure heart failure. If medical therapy is not adequate to decrease the LA pressure, a fenestrated ASD closure device can be used to avoid the development of acute left heart failure.

IMAGING OF IAS AND SEPTAL DEFECTS

Patent foramen ovale

The occurrence of a PFO is common, present in 20–25% of the population, and the anatomy has been extensively discussed earlier in the present document. PFO has been associated with cryptogenic stroke, decompression sickness, platypnea-orthodeoxia syndrome and migraine headache. Controversy exists regarding the role of PFO in these syndromes, and currently, transcatheter procedures to close the PFO in an attempt to decrease the incidence of these problems are not approved. Echocardiography has a central role in the evaluation of PFO and monitoring/guidance of PFO closure, similar to its role in ASD closure. A TTE evaluation of PFO, including the use of agitated saline contrast, is primarily used to identify the presence or absence of a PFO according to the presence or absence of right-to-left shunting. Once a PFO has been identified, and percutaneous device closure is being considered, a detailed evaluation of the atrial septal anatomy is performed using TEE. TEE can also be used if a PFO is suspected; however, TTE is technically inadequate to rule out the presence of a PFO. The TEE views used for the evaluation of a PFO are similar to those used for the evaluation of an ASD. Starting in the transverse plane at the midesophagus, with settings optimized to visualize the atrial septum, the TEE imaging plane should be rotated or steered, starting at a 0° multiplane angle, in 15° increments, for complete evaluation of the atrial septum. Side-by-side imaging with colour Doppler at a low colour Doppler scale is helpful for identifying flow through the PFO and possible additional defects in the atrial septum. The probe will need to be withdrawn for better evaluation of the atrial septum near the SVC and inserted for better evaluation of the atrial septum near the IVC. Alternatively, an initial evaluation of the atrial septum can be performed in the transverse plane, starting at the high esophageal level at the SVC and advancing the probe in the oesophagus, imaging through the fossa ovalis and ending at the level of the IVC. A similar manoeuvre can be performed with the imaging plane at 90°–120°.

Starting at 30°–50°, with the AoV in cross section, the PFO should be visualized adjacent to the aorta. Rotation of the imaging plane in 15° increments should align the imaging plane with the pathway or tunnel of the PFO. From this angle, the length of the PFO tunnel can be assessed. The thickness of the septum secundum can also be evaluated from this view. With the PFO visualized, agitated saline contrast is injected to evaluate for right-to-left shunting, as described in the section 'Techniques, characterization, standards and visualization of shunting: TTE and TEE'.[12] Provocative manoeuvres such as the Valsalva manoeuvre should be performed for adequate assessment so as to transiently increase the RA pressure over the LA pressure.

Important anatomic details of the atrial septum that should be evaluated because they can influence device candidacy and selection include the location of the PFO (although, unlike secundum ASD, the location of a PFO is fairly consistent in the anterior or superior portion of the fossa ovalis), thickness and extent of septum secundum, total length of the atrial septum, length of the PFO tunnel, size of the PFO at the RA and LA ends, distance of the PFO from the venae cavae, presence of ASA and presence of additional atrial septal fenestrations or defects. As with ASD, partial anomalous pulmonary venous connection should be excluded. Real-time 3D (RT3D) TEE has been used to better define PFO variations compared with 2D TEE. RT3D TEE has shown that the shape of the PFO is elliptical, not circular, and that the flow area decreases traversing from the RA to the LA. As with secundum ASD, the area of the PFO changes during the cardiac cycle and is larger during ventricular systole than diastole. RT3D TEE has also been used for procedural guidance of closure with en face views of the atrial septum showing the relationship of the PFO and device with the surrounding structures in the RA and LA (Figure 4.32).

Specific anatomic characteristics of a PFO should be evaluated when deciding on device selection for PFO closure. Specifically, the diameter of the fossa ovalis, length of the PFO tunnel, presence and size of an ASA, thickness of the septum secundum and maximum size of the PFO during the cardiac cycle are all important in appropriate patient selection for transcatheter closure.

An ASA is a redundancy or saccular deformity of the atrial septum associated with increased mobility (Figure 4.21). An ASA is defined as an excursion of 10 mm from the plane of the atrial septum into the RA or LA or a combined excursion right and left of 15 mm.[17] M-mode can be used to document this motion when the cursor can be aligned perpendicular to the plane of the septum[16] (Figure 4.34). A more detailed classification system (that has not been widely clinically adopted) has divided ASAs into five groups based on the excursion exclusively into the RA or LA, predominantly into the RA or LA, or with equal excursion right and left.[18] ASA has been associated with the presence of a PFO or ASD, an increased size of a PFO and an increased prevalence of cryptogenic stroke and other embolic events. ASA has also been associated with multiple septal fenestrations. TEE is a more sensitive method than TTE for evaluation of an ASA. The presence and extent of an ASA is a factor in device selection for PFO closure. A device can be chosen that is relatively large to encompass and

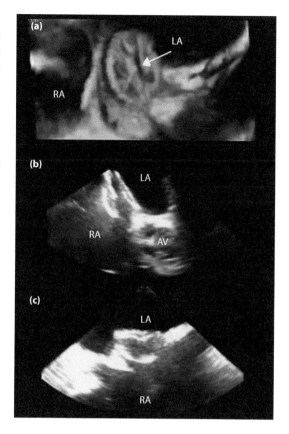

Figure 4.32 Triplane of cribriform closure device deployed during PFO closure: 3D (a), biplane orthogonal short-axis (b) and biplane orthogonal long-axis views (c). The yellow arrow specifies LA disc of closure device. AV, aortic valve. (Adapted from ASE guidelines for echocardiographic assessment of ASD and PFO, August 2015.)

stabilize the atrial septum or a smaller and softer device might be chosen for better conformation with the ASA.[19] The excursion of the atrial septum can be documented using 2D imaging as well as M-mode assessment when the M-mode cursor can be aligned perpendicular to the plane of the IAS. This can be done in the subcostal four-chamber view on TTE, in the bicaval views on TEE and in the septal long-axis views on ICE (Figure 4.33).

The Eustachian valve extends anteriorly from the IVC–RA junction and is best visualized on TTE from the subxiphoid coronal and sagittal views. On TEE, the Eustachian valve is best visualized in the longitudinal plane. The size of the Eustachian valve and proximity to the IAS should be noted on the echocardiographic evaluation, because a large Eustachian valve that is close to

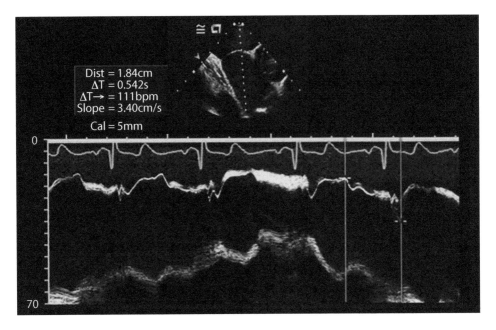

Figure 4.33 M-mode of an ASA demonstrating greater than 15 mm mobility of the fossa on ICE imaging. Eustachian valve and Chiari network. (Adapted from ASE guidelines for echocardiographic assessment of ASD and PFO, August 2015.)

the IAS can interfere in the deployment of the RA side of a closure device.[20] A Chiari network is a remnant of the right valve of the sinus venosus and appears as a filamentous structure in various places in the RA, including near the mouth of the IVC and coronary sinus (Figure 4.34). A Chiari network can interfere in the passage through the RA of wires, catheters, sheaths, cables and the device. Therefore, the identification of the presence of a Chiari network should be a part of the echocardiographic evaluation before device closure of an ASD or a PFO.[21]

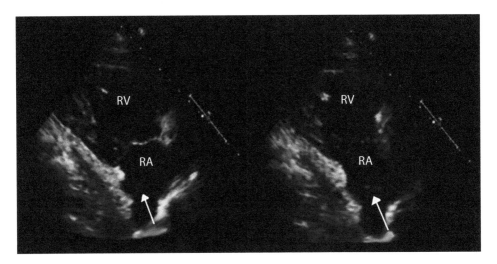

Figure 4.34 Transthoracic echocardiogram from the RV inflow view demonstrating mobile Chiari network (white arrows) attached to Eustachian ridge. (Adapted from ASE guidelines for echocardiographic assessment of ASD and PFO, August 2015.)

REFERENCES

1. Silvestry FE, Cohen MS, Armsby LB, et al. Guidelines for the echocardiographic assessment of atrial septal defect and patent foramen ovale: From the American Society of Echocardiography and Society for Cardiac Angiography and Interventions. *J Am Soc Echocardiogr.* 2015; 28(8):910–958.

2. Hahn RT, Abraham T, Adams MS, et al. Guidelines for performing a comprehensive transesophageal echocardiographic examination: Recommendations from the American Society of Echocardiography and the Society of Cardiovascular Anesthesiologists. *J Am Soc Echocardiogr.* 2013; 26:921–964.

3. Lang RMR, Badano LPL, Tsang WW, et al. EAE/ASE recommendations for image acquisition and display using three-dimensional echocardiography. *J Am Soc Echocardiogr.* 2012; 25:3–46.

4. Yared K, Baggish AL, Solis J, et al. Echocardiographic assessment of percutaneous patent foramen ovale and atrial septal defect closure complications. *Circ Cardiovasc Imaging.* 2009; 2:141–149.

5. Rosenzweig BP, Nayar AC, Varkey MP, Kronzon I. Echo contrast enhanced diagnosis of atrial septal defect. *J Am Soc Echocardiogr.* 2001; 14:155–157.

6. Bartel T, Muller S. Device closure of inter-atrial communications: Peri-interventional echocardiographic assessment. *Eur Heart J Cardiovasc Imaging.* 2013; 14:618–624.

7. Taniguchi M, Akagi T, Watanabe N, et al. Application of real-time three-dimensional transesophageal echocardiography using a matrix array probe for trans catheter closure of atrial septal defect. *J Am Soc Echocardiogr.* 2009; 22:1114–1120.

8. Bhan A, Kapetanakis S, Pearson P, Dworakowski R, Monaghan MJ. Percutaneous closure of an atrial septal defect guided by live three dimensional transesophageal echocardiography. *J Am Soc Echocardiogr.* 2009; 22:753.e1–3.

9. Belkin RN, Pollack BD, Ruggiero ML, Alas LL, Tatini U. Comparison of transesophageal and transthoracic echocardiography with contrast and color flow Doppler in the detection of patent foramen ovale. *Am Heart J.* 1994; 128:520–525.

10. Vigna C, Marchese N, Zanchetta M, et al. Echocardiographic guidance of percutaneous patent foramen ovale closure: Head-to-head comparison of transesophageal versus rotational intracardiac echocardiography. *Echocardiography.* 2012; 29:1103–1110.

11. Thanigaraj S, Valika A, Zajarias A, Lasala JM, Perez JE. Comparison of transthoracic versus transesophageal echocardiography for detection of right-to-left atrial shunting using agitated saline contrast. *Am J Cardiol.* 2005; 96:1007–1010.

12. Woods TD, Patel A. A critical review of patent foramen ovale detection using saline contrast echocardiography: When bubbles lie. *J Am Soc Echocardiogr.* 2006; 19:215–222.

13. Soliman OII, Geleijnse ML, Meijboom FJ, et al. The use of contrast echocardiography for the detection of cardiac shunts. *Eur J Echocardiogr.* 2007; 8:S2–12.

14. Corrado G, Massironi L, Torta D, et al. Contrast transthoracic echocardiography versus transcranial Doppler for patent foramen ovale detection. *Int J Cardiol.* 2011; 150:235–237.

15. Draganski B, Blersch W, Holmer S, et al. Detection of cardiac right-to-left shunts by contrast-enhanced harmonic carotid duplex sonography. *J Ultrasound Med.* 2005; 24:1071–1076.

16. Topçuoglu MA, Palacios IF, Buonanno FS, et al. Contrast M-mode power Doppler ultrasound in the detection of right-to-left shunts: Utility of submandibular internal carotid artery recording. *J Neuroimaging.* 2003; 13(4):315–323.

17. Agmon Y, Khandheria BK, Meissner I, et al. Frequency of atrial septal aneurysms in patients with cerebral ischemic events. *Circulation.* 1999; 99:1942–1944.

18. Giannopoulos A, Gavras C, Sarioglou S, Agathagelou F, Kassapoglou I, Athanassiadou F. Atrial septal aneurysms in childhood: Prevalence, classification, and concurrent abnormalities. *Cardiol Young.* 2014; 24:453–458.

19. Krumsdorf U, Keppeler P, Horvath K, Zadan E, Schrader R, Sievert H. Catheter closure of atrial septal defects and patent foramen ovale in patients with an atrial septal aneurysm using different devices. *J Interv Cardiol.* 2001; 14:49–55.

20. Schuchlenz HW, Saurer G, Weihs W, Rehak P. Persisting Eustachian valve in adults: Relation to patent foramen ovale and cerebrovascular events. *J Am Soc Echocardiogr.* 2004; 17:231–233.

21. Schneider B, Hofmann T, Justen MH, Meinertz T. Chiari's network: Normal anatomic variant or risk factor for arterial embolic events. *J Am Coll Cardiol.* 1995; 26:203–210.

Assessment of morphology of defects: Standards and characterization

A A PILLAI

Atrial septal defects (ASDs) represent a diverse group of differing anatomic lesions that all result in intracardiac shunting. The common features of all ASD types that should be systematically evaluated and reported for all ASD types are listed in Table 5.1. These include the type of ASD (primum or secundum) or other atrial communication (venosus or unroofed coronary sinus); the presence and direction of Doppler flow through the defect; and associated findings such as anomalous pulmonary vein drainage, the presence and size of a Eustachian valve or a Chiari network, the size and shape of the defect or defects, the location in the septum, the presence or absence of multiple fenestrations and the size of the ASD at end-systole and end-diastole. Ostium secundum ASD is the most common defect encountered and most commonly occurs as a deficiency in septum primum. Secundum ASDs can vary considerably in their size, shape and configuration, as has been described previously. A small ASD is typically described as less than 5 mm in the maximal measured ASD diameter. With favourable anatomic features, ostium secundum ASDs can be amenable to percutaneous transcatheter closure. Secundum ASDs have a variable amount of surrounding tissue that borders the defect, and these 'rims' of surrounding tissue are named for the corresponding surrounding adjacent anatomic structures. By convention, there are six anatomically named rims of surrounding tissue. These rims should be assessed carefully, using echocardiography in all patients and, in particular, before consideration of percutaneous closure. A rim length of 5 mm or more is considered a favourable characteristic for percutaneous transcatheter closure of a secundum ASD. An ASD rim length of less than 5 mm is described as 'deficient' and could present challenges for transcatheter closure.[1] Secundum ASD rims can be defined as follows:

1. **Aortic rim:** the superior/anterior rim between the ASD and the AoV annulus and aortic root
2. **AV valve rim**: the inferior/anterior rim between the ASD and the AV valves
3. **SVC rim**: the superior/posterior rim between the ASD and the SVC
4. **IVC rim**: the inferior/posterior rim between the ASD and the IVC
5. **Posterior rim**: the posterior rim between ASD and posterior atrial walls
6. **Right upper pulmonary vein (RUPV) rim**: the posterior rim between the ASD and the RUPV

Having adequate superior, inferior and anterior rims (SVC, RUPV, IVC and AV valve rims) is particularly important for successful transcatheter ASD closure. A deficient aortic rim has been

Table 5.1 Specific characteristics of ASD that should be routinely measured and reported

ASD type—PFO, primum ASD, secundum ASD or other atrial communication (sinus venosus defect, unroofed coronary sinus, anomalous pulmonary vein drainage)

Doppler flow—presence of left-to-right, right-to-left or bidirectional flow

Presence or absence of atrial septal aneurysm

Associated findings—Eustachian valve or Chiari network

ASD size—maximal and minimal diameters (best measured from 3D volume data images)

ASD area

ASD location in septum (i.e., high secundum ASD, sinus venosus defect SVC or IVC type)

Measurement of all rims—aortic, RUPV, AV septal, superior, posterior, inferior.

Shape of ASD—round, oval, irregular

Presence of multiple fenestrations

Dynamic nature of ASD—measurement of area and maximum/minimal diameters in end-systole and end-diastole images

Stop-flow diameter of ASD (can be measured when balloon sizing is used for percutaneous trans catheter closure)

---

implicated as a potential risk factor for erosion, although it might not represent an absolute contraindication to device closure.[2] Transesophageal echocardiography (TEE) evaluates these six ASD rims in the upper oesophageal short-axis, midesophageal short-axis, four-chamber and bicaval views, and transthoracic echocardiography (TTE) provides similar views. The TEE views and corresponding rims evaluated are listed in Table 5.1. Although TTE might be adequate for the evaluation of rims in smaller paediatric patients, in larger paediatric and adult patients, it will typically be inadequate. Therefore, TEE is recommended for these patients to assess these rims before transcatheter closure.[3] Intracardiac echocardiographic (ICE) has been demonstrated to provide images of the ASD rims similar to those with TEE, although no true four-chamber view is possible with ICE. TEE with 3D imaging, if available, should be considered for all patients under consideration for percutaneous closure—even if an ICE-guided closure procedure is being planned.

REFERENCES

1. Amin Z. Transcatheter closure of secundum atrial septal defects. *Catheter Cardiovasc Interv.* 2006; 68(5):778–787.
2. Ananthakrishna Pillai A, Sinouvassalou S, Jagadessan KS, Munuswamy H. Spectrum of morphological abnormalities and treatment outcomes in ostium secundum type of atrial septal defects: Single center experience in >500 cases. *J Saudi Heart Assoc.* 2019; 31(1):12–23. 10.1016/j.jsha.2018.09.002.
3. Bartel T, Müller S. Device closure of interatrial communications: Peri-interventional assessment. *Eur Heart J Cardiovasc Imaging.* 2013; 14:618–624.

Indications of ASD closure

A A PILLAI, A HANDA

The American College of Cardiology/American Heart Association guidelines have recommended atrial septal defect (ASD) closure for patients with right atrial (RA) and right ventricular (RV) enlargement, regardless of symptoms (class I). Small ASDs (i.e., an ASD diameter of less than 5 mm) with no evidence of RV enlargement or pulmonary hypertension do not require closure because they are not considered significant enough to affect the clinical course or haemodynamics of these individuals. Smaller ASDs that are associated with paradoxical embolism or platypnea-orthodeoxia can be considered for closure according to guideline recommendations (class IIa). The only absolute contraindication for ASD closure pertains to patients with irreversible pulmonary hypertension (pulmonary vascular resistance greater than 8 Woods units) and no evidence of left-to-right shunting (class III). Sinus venosus and ostium primum defects are not suitable for percutaneous device closure because of poor anatomic and rim characteristics and the lack of randomized controlled trial data supporting this approach. The indications and contraindications to ASD and PFO closure are listed in Table 6.1.[1]

Numerous devices exist for percutaneous transcatheter closure of ASDs and PFOs (Figure 6.1). The Amplatzer and the Gore PFO occlusion systems are approved by the US FDA for the percutaneous transcatheter closure of PFOs. The two types of devices currently approved in the United States for transcatheter closure of secundum ASDs are the Helex (W.L.Gore, Newark, DE) and Amplatzer (St. Jude Medical, Plymouth, MN) septal occlude devices[2] (Figure 6.1). Only secundum ASDs have been approved by the FDA to be treated with these percutaneous transcatheter closure devices. Thus, patients with sinus venosus and primum defects should be evaluated for surgical repair, if appropriate. The Helex occluder (W.L. Gore) is composed of expanded poly tetrafluoroethylene patch material supported by a single nitinol wire frame. The device bridges and eventually occludes the septal defect as cells infiltrate and ultimately cover the expanded poly tetrafluoroethylene membrane. The Helex occluder (W.L. Gore) is not recommended for closure of defects larger than 18 mm in diameter or those in which the rim is absent over more than 25% of the circumference of the defect. The Amplatzer septal occluder (ASO) and Amplatzer multifenestrated cribriform septal occluder (St. Jude Medical) are double-disc devices composed of nitinol mesh and polyester fabric. These devices are designed to appose the septal wall on each side of the defect, creating a platform for tissue ingrowth after implantation. The ASO (St. Jude Medical) is a self-centring device with a waist sized to fill the diameter of a single ASD. The narrow waist of the cribriform device is specifically designed to allow placement through the central defect of a fenestrated septum; the matched disc diameters positioned on either side of the septum

Table 6.1 Indications and contraindications for ASD and PFO closure

Potential Indications for ASD and PFO closure

- Isolated secundum ASD with a pulmonary/systemic flow (Qp/Qs) ratio 1.5:1, signs of right ventricular volume overload
- PFO—cryptogenic stroke and evidence of right-to-left shunt

Contraindications (absolute or relative)

- PFO or small ASD with Qp/Qs <1.5:1 or no signs of RV volume overload
- A single defect too large for closure (>38 mm)
- Multiple ASDs unsuitable for percutaneous closure
- Defect too close to superior vena cava (SVC), inferior vena cava (IVC), pulmonary veins, AV valves or coronary sinus
- Anterior, posterior, superior or inferior rim <5 mm
- Abnormal pulmonary venous drainage
- Associated congenital abnormality requiring cardiac surgery
- ASD with severe pulmonary arterial hypertension and bidirectional or right-to-left shunting intracardiac thrombi diagnosed by echocardiography

maximize coverage of multiple fenestrations. The ASO (St. Jude Medical) is contraindicated in patients in whom a deficiency (defined as less than 5 mm) of septal rim is present between the defect and the right pulmonary vein, AV valve or IVC. Although a deficiency of the aortic rim is not considered an absolute contraindication to the use of the device, it has been suggested that this could increase the risk of device erosion. A significant proportion of defects are associated with absent or deficient aortic rims, and although erosion after ASD device closure occurs most often in these patients, the great majority of these defects can be successfully closed by a device without subsequent

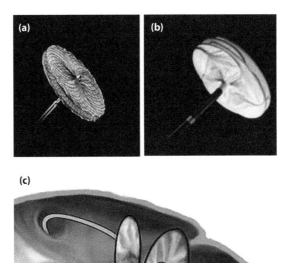

Figure 6.1 Examples of ASD closure devices. ASO (St. Jude Medical) (a). Helex occluder (W.L. Gore) (b). Deployment of ASD device (c): 4C, four-chamber (view); Ao, aorta; SAX, short-axis (view). (Illustration by Saranya Gousy.)

erosion. The Helex septal occluders (W.L. Gore) and ASOs (St. Jude Medical) are deployed using their unique delivery systems by way of venous access after careful assessment of the atrial septum and sizing of the defect.

DEVICE EMBOLIZATION AND EROSION

Complications of percutaneous PFO and ASD closure devices are rare and include device embolization, cardiac perforation, tamponade and device erosion. Device embolization occurs in approximately 0.1–0.4% of cases, particularly with ASD closure devices. Device embolization is a potentially life-threatening complication requiring immediate removal by either percutaneous or surgical intervention. Device embolization can be readily diagnosed by routine surveillance TTE. The risk factors for device embolization include an undersized ASD device, deficient rims of surrounding tissue and device malpositioning. Immediate embolization can occur after device deployment and most likely results from device malpositioning or an incorrect device size. TTE and TEE are invaluable tools in evaluating the precise location of a dislodged device and the physiologic sequelae (e.g., inflow/outflow obstruction, valve disruption) that result from the embolization.

Device erosion is a rare but potentially fatal event. Erosion has been reported to occur with multiple devices, including the ASO (St. Jude Medical), the atrial septal defect occluder system and the Angel-Wings device (Microvena Corp., White Bear Lake, MN). Of these, only the ASO (St. Jude Medical) is currently approved for use in the United States. The estimated rate of erosion with the ASO (St. Jude Medical) is 0.1–0.3%. Device erosion can occur at the roof of the RA or LA or at the junction of the aorta and can result in haemopericardium, tamponade, aortic fistula and/or death. Device erosion can begin as a subclinical event, with the device impinging on the surrounding structures, tenting the atrial or aortic tissue or resulting in a subclinical pericardial effusion. Erosion can also manifest clinically with chest pain, syncope, shortness of breath, the development of a haemopericardium, cardiac tamponade, haemodynamic compromise and death. Most cases of erosion have been reported to occur within 72 hours of device implantation, but late erosion

cases have been reported more than 6 years after deployment. Most erosions occur in the first week after implantation. Although the cause is not well defined, it has been assumed that erosion is related to the abrasive mechanical forces between the human tissue and the device (in contrast to inflammation). The cause of erosions is unknown. A thorough understanding of this serious problem has been hampered by the infrequency of this complication and the absence of data from control populations. Extensive reviews of imaging and device data from series of cases in which erosions occurred have been performed. From such information and expert consensus, the factors can be broadly divided into those generally thought to be more significant, such as device oversizing (present in up to 40% of cases), the complete absence of the aortic rim, a high/superior septal location of the defect and a deficient anterior rim with associated insufficiency of the posterior rim. Other morphologic risk factors that have been proposed to predict erosion include a specific ASD orientation such as malalignment of the defect with the aorta, a dynamic ASD (one that changes size more than 50% throughout the cardiac cycle), a deficient or an absent aortic rim (present in up to 90% of cases) and a device that straddles or splays around the aorta. No consensus has been reached, however, in the interventional community regarding the root cause of erosion. It is important to note, for example, that a deficient aortic rim is prevalent among populations of patients who have undergone successful device closure of ASD with the ASO (St. Jude Medical) (40% in a recent report). Important risk factors for erosion after device placement have been suggested from a retrospective review of available data on confirmed cases and include deformation of the closure device at the aortic root and pericardial effusion seen within 24 hours of deployment. The proposed risk factors for erosion of the Amplatzer device are listed in Table 6.2. No one risk factor or echocardiographic feature can absolutely define the absolute risk for device erosion. Thus, there are no clear echocardiographic contraindications for device closure. In one conceptual framework, for example, erosion might result from the unique combination of certain specific high-risk ASD morphologic features that are then combined with an oversized device and subsequent remodelling of the heart and closure device. Echocardiographic imaging therefore

Table 6.2 Proposed possible risk factors for Amplatzer device erosion

- Deficient aortic rim in multiple views, absent aortic rim at 0° referred to as bald aorta
- Deficient superior rim in multiple views
- Superior location of secundum ASD
- Oversized ASD device (device diameter >1.5 times static stop-flow diameter)
- Dynamic ASD (50% change in size of ASD)
- Use of 26-mm ASO device
- Malaligned defect
- Tenting of atrial septal free wall after placement of device (into transverse sinus)
- Wedging of device disc between posterior wall and aorta
- Pericardial effusion present after device placement

might help to identify patients at risk of erosion (e.g., aortic rim deficiencies, device–patient mismatch at the atrial roof, or impingement of the aorta before release). The FDA and the manufacturer have concurred that an additional post-approval study of the ASO (St. Jude Medical) would be beneficial to better evaluate the risk factors for erosion. A standardized rigorous protocol for the evaluation of the atrial septum and associated rims, such as described in the present document, has the potential to increase the quality and consistency of the data used to analyze the root cause and prevent this rare, but serious, complication.

Newer Figulla Flex (Occlutech) devices marketed with CE marking claim superior alignment on account of tilted disc arrangement favouring the deficient aortic rim. However, the experience in using this device is growing. Bioabsorbable devices are the next frontier in the pipeline. These may be applicable in small defects in which the devices (magnesium alloy) will be reabsorbed within 18–24 months, similar to bio reabsorbable stents. The defect will be closed by the endothelial layer that forms over the device over time.

REFERENCES

1. Warnes CA, Williams RG, Bashore TM, et al. ACC/AHA 2008 guidelines for the management of adults with congenital heart disease: A report of the American College of Cardiology/American Heart Association task force on practice guidelines (writing committee to develop guidelines on the management of adults with congenital heart disease). Developed in collaboration with the American Society of Echocardiography, Heart Rhythm Society, International Society for Adult Congenital Heart Disease, Society for Cardiovascular Angiography and Interventions, and Society of Thoracic surgeons. *J Am Coll Cardiol*. 2008; 52(23):e143–e263.
2. Bennhagen RG, McLaughlin P, Benson LN. CardioSeal and StarFlex devices. In Rao PS, Kern MJ, editors. Catheter based devices for treatment of noncoronary cardiovascular disease in adults and children. Philadelphia (PA): Lippincott, Williams & Wilkins; 2003; 61–69.

7

ASD closure devices: History and present

V BALASUBRAMANIAN

Atrial septal defects (ASDs) are the most common congenital heart defects in adults and second most common in children after ventricular septal defects. Unrepaired ASDs can lead to significant mortality and morbidity. Of the various types of ASD, only secundum ASD can be closed by percutaneous methods. Since 1952, surgical ASD closure was the only treatment available for patients with ASD until percutaneous ASD closure was introduced by King and Mills in 1975.[4] Transcatheter closure outperformed surgical closure in early mortality, complications such as embolization, atrial fibrillation and thromboembolism.[3] Continued development has been incorporated in the device designs, which has made percutaneous closure the current treatment of choice in most secundum ASD cases.[1,2] Transcatheter technology is a maturing technology and has been regarded as safe and effective. Observational studies have shown percutaneous device closure outperforming surgical repair with lower rates of complications.[2] To accommodate the required technical refinements, many device changes have taken place in the last four decades. Some of the devices were discontinued due to technical reasons. We present the history of development of ASD devices over last four decades in this review.[1,2]

Since the first ASD device by King and Mills in 1975, a number of devices were developed, but only few of them reached clinical usage. The following devices were significant in the history of ASD devices.[2,4]

1. King and Mills cardiac umbrella
2. Rashkind single umbrella
3. Lock Clamshell Occluder
4. Sideris buttoned device
5. Atrial septal defect occluding system
6. Monodisk (Pavcnik's)
7. Angel Wings
8. CardioSEAL and STAR flex
9. Solysafe Septal Occluder

Food and Drug Administration (FDA)–approved devices in clinical use

1. Amplatzer Septal Occluder (ASO)—current gold standard
2. GORE HELEX Cardioform Septal Occluder

CE-approved devices in clinical use

1. Occlutech Figulla (Flex) Occluder
2. Lifetech Cera ASD occluder and CeraFlex ASD occluder
3. Cardio Atriasept I/II and Ultracept I/II
4. Nitocclud ASD-R (NOASD-R)

Bioresorbable septal occludes devices

1. BioSTAR and BioTREK (discontinued)
2. Immediate-release patch (IRP)
3. Carag Bioresorbable Septal Occluder (CBSO).

Pioneering works of King and Mills in 1975 paved way for ASD closure devices and more than 20 devices have been developed till now, of which 12 have been discontinued and 8 of them currently have FDA (or) CE approval. Over the last four decades, closure devices have become lighter; less material for enhancing endothelialisation and a smaller delivery sheath have improved ASD closure technique, which has led to attempting percutaneous device closure in complex ASD defects also. An ideal device requires completes defect closure with no complications. None of the currently available devices satisfies that criterion. Future developments like wireless bioresorbable devices

can reduce complications related to hardware. If bioresorbable devices are successful, they will provide a breakthrough in the development of percutaneous ASD closure devices.

KING AND MILLS CARDIAC UMBRELLA

King and Mills were the first to introduce percutaneous closure technique for atrial septal defect when they designed a closure device which was first implanted in dogs in 1972.[4] This device was made of paired Dacron-covered stainless steel umbrellas collapsed into a capsule at the tip of a catheter. ASD closure was initially attempted in dogs by punching atrial septal defects, and complete closure of ASD and endothelialisation was noted during follow-up. Following experience in canine models this technique was extended to human studies.[5] Stretched ASD diameter was measured by sizing balloon and a device larger than 10 mm of stretched diameter was deployed. The device was delivered through femoral venous cut down. The catheter tip was positioned in left atrium through ASD. The device is extruded in left atrium and catheter withdrawn into right atrium. The distal umbrella is fixed against left atrial side and right-sided umbrella deployed in right atrial side of septum with a special locking mechanism both umbrellas were fixed. Then obturator wire is withdrawn releasing the device. Successful implantation was done in 50% of patients.[5] Later with help of Edward laboratories, some modifications were made and the device was successfully implanted in humans in 1975. It was a paired umbrella-type device with six stainless steel struts ending in hooks. Despite initial positive results, the device was not used again due to lack of self-centring and irretrievability and the need for surgical removal in case of suboptimal device placement. Also requirement of large sheaths of 23 F due to a bulky device and complex manoeuvrability did not help. However, the King and Mills device paved the way for newer technology in ASD devices.

RASHKIND SINGLE UMBRELLA

Almost at the same time of King and Mills work, Rashkind developed a different type of ASD device which had a single umbrella consisting of medical grade foam covered with three stainless steel ribs attached to central hub.[6] He modified it into six ribbed device with three hooks attached to alternate ribs. The central hub was attached to 6-F catheter. The umbrella was held by five arms on the tip of guide wire. Rashkind's device did have a centring mechanism and, by retracting the guidewire through the septal defect, its five arms could bend to produce an outward curve. The umbrella bends and hooks onto the left atrial side of the septum and, by further retracting the guidewire, the delivery system unlocks from the umbrella. This centring mechanism required a 14-F (or) 16-F sheath. After encouraging animal experiments, this device was deployed in 23 patients in whom only 60% was successful. Due to poor outcomes Rashkind developed a double umbrella version of the device, but, pending clinical trials, the device did not reach clinical use. Several disadvantages, such as the requirement of a large sheath and instantaneously permanent positioning due to anchoring hooks and the inability to reposition, might have discouraged further use. Sometimes the device got attached to mitral valve, requiring surgical intervention. Also complete endothelialization and damage to adjacent structures after successful implantation requiring surgical intervention discouraged its use. But the double-disc version was picked up by other investigators, and after further modifications the device was renamed as Lock Clamshell Occluder.

LOCK CLAMSHELL OCCLUDER (CR BARD INC, MURRAY HILL)

Lock et al., co-investigators in the development of Rashkind double umbrella, made certain modifications with a spring in the middle of all four umbrella arms and renamed it as the Lock Clamshell Occluder device.[2] These springs helped by holding both umbrellas against each other, producing clamshell-like appearance. The device was made of non-hooked stainless steel frame covered with Dacron and delivered through an 11-F sheath. Although device had technical improvement and retrievability, 40–84% of them had arm fractures, device embolization, residual shunt and new stroke. Hence it went out of clinical use. Later device was modified due to proven

superiority compared with older devices. The device was modified into CardioSEAL and then later STARFlex.

BUTTONED DEVICE (CUSTOM MEDICAL DEVICES, ATHENS, GREECE)

Sideris et al. introduced buttoned ASD device in 1990.[13] A number of modifications led to four generations of left-sided occluders and counter occluders with different shapes. The button occluder was a squared polyurethane disc with an x-shaped Teflon-coated stainless steel frame and a button that is a loop knot and counter occluder containing buttonhole and Teflon-coated steel wire in its foam disc. When both discs were deployed, a button on left atrial side was pulled through right-side button hole to connect them. The device required an 8-F to 9-F loading sheath. None of the four generations of devices had self-centring mechanism. Hence a centring mechanism introduced because of demand. Effective closure was achieved in 90% defects, as the device got pulled through in cases of large defects. Extensive single and multiple clinical trials were done between 1990 and 2001, and the buttoned device was found feasible and effective in closing atrial septal defects. Initial implantations were done in piglets and later in humans. During initial implantation in a child, after buttoning the device during deployment, it spontaneously dislodged due to tearing of the tie between the occluder and counter occluder due to excessive force used while buttoning. The first three generation of devices had a problem of unbuttoning post-procedure and subsequent surgical retrieval. This led to device modification, replacing silk tie with nylon tie and a radio-opaque marker on the button so that no excessive force can be used while buttoning. Further refinements were made, such as incorporation of additional nylon thread, reducing eccentricity of the buttoning and converting it into a straight one; this improved fourth-generation version could be directly loaded onto the delivery sheath, and an over-the-wire delivery technique was developed. Despite incidents of fewer unbuttoning and fewer residual shunts, these problems were a cause of concern. Despite widespread clinical experience, the device never received FDA approval and was discontinued.

ATRIAL SEPTAL DEFECT OCCLUDER SYSTEM (GERMANY)

A European ASD closure device called an atrial septal defect occluding system (ASDOS) 2001 was developed in 1990 by Babic et al. Device went through several modifications and finally got licensed in 1994.[7] Two separate umbrellas with polyurethane frames and nitinol arms were implanted through an 11-F sheath by forming an arterio-venous loop. The first umbrella deployed in the left atrium. A metal plug was used to prevent distal migration and for centring the device, after which it was pulled into right atrium. Another catheter with a screw mechanism was used to deploy the second umbrella. Two umbrellas were screwed after correct positioning using a metal plug. Despite obtaining CE approval in 1995, the device was abandoned in 2001 in view of high incidence of frame fractures, Thrombus formation and atrial wall perforation. However, introduction of nitinol frame led to era of devices with reduced risk of fracture and ability to reshape after deployment.

NITINOL DEVICES— TECHNOLOGICAL LEAP

In 1962 William Buehler (US Naval Labs) found that an alloy containing equal amounts of nickel and titanium exhibited a strange character which allowed catheter-based devices to take a big step forward. The property of assuming a distorted shape inside the delivery catheter and regaining the preformed shape when deployed led to its use for ASD closure. These alloy materials have proven useful in devices with better centring characteristics and considerably lesser risk of stress fractures. This is considered a technological leap with unlimited boundaries in device engineering.

MONODISK

Pavcnik et al. (1993) designed a Monodisk[8] (Figure 7.1) consisting of a single disc of stainless steel rings constructed from spring coil wire covered by double-layered nylon mesh with three hollow pieces of stainless steel wires sutured onto the right side of the device. Three strands of monofilament nylon pass through each of the hollow wires. The nylon thread passes through the delivery catheter. The entire device can be loaded over

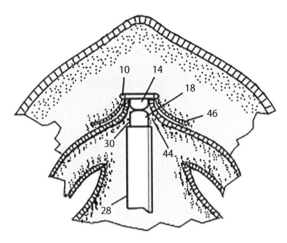

Figure 7.1 Pavcnik's monodisk. (Illustration by Saranya Gousy.)

9-F sheath. Once the device was positioned it was deployed by cutting the wires. The device was successfully implanted in dogs and subsequently in two patients. But no clinical trials were planned and pending long-term studies the device was discontinued. Pavcnik further introduced a modified version like a biodisc and double biodisc, but it fell out of favour for unknown reasons.

MODIFIED RASHKIND PDA UMBRELLA DEVICE

The Rashkind PDA umbrella device was modified by bending the arms of the device such that there is better apposition of the device to the atrial septum. The device was used to close four ASDs, two of which were removed with subsequent surgical closure. The use of this device for ASD closure was questioned and subsequently went out of use.

ANGEL WINGS (MICROVENA CORP, WHITE BEAR LAKE, MINNESOTA, USA)

In 1993 Das et al. developed a new device called the DAS Angel Wings device which had two polyester fabric-covered square frames and a nitinol frame with mid-point torsion spring eyelets.[11] The nitinol frame served as a torsion spring to provide a folding mechanism. A circular hole with a diameter equal to one-half the size of the disc was punched from right disc, with the margins sewn to left disc forming a conjoined ring, the centring mechanism. Device sizes ranged from 12 to 40 mm and were delivered transvenously through 11-F or 12-F sheath. Most device required 12-F sheath. Device did not cross phase II trials and was modified to become the Guardian Angel Wings device, but the device was shelved. Device malpositioning during deployment was the main reason for its discontinuation.

CARDIOSEAL AND STARFLEX

The Lock clamshell device was discontinued due to breakage of arms due to stress fractures and was redesigned by replacing stainless steel of the umbrella arms with MP35N, a nonferrous alloy, and by introducing additional bends in the arms of the device. It was renamed as CardioSEAL[14] in 1996 (Ryan et al.). Further modification was made by introducing a self-centring mechanism by attaching microsprings between umbrellas, and it was named STARFlex in 1999 (Hausdorf et al.).

Both these devices were tested in European multicentre trials conducted from October 1996 to April 1999. Device implantation was done in 334 patients with success in 325 patients. Device to balloon stretched diameter was two times more. Embolization occurred shortly in 13 patients, of which 10 underwent surgical retrieval and the remaining 3 had catheter removal. Residual shunts were seen in 41% immediately after the procedure which reduced to 21% at 12 months.[15] Both devices were used to close small to moderate sized defects. They were not suitable for closing large or complex defects.

STARFlex was further modified as BioSTAR and BioTREK with bioabsorbable materials.

GORE HELEX/CARDIO FORM SEPTAL OCCLUDER

The Helex Septal Occluder (HSO) is a non-self-centring device made of a single, spring-like nitinol frame wire covered by an ultrathin expanded polytetrafluoroethylene membrane.[16] This flexible frame is stretched around a central axis which is delivered through a 9-F sheath. The central locking system is the only uncovered metal of the device to minimize exposure to blood. The first implantation in humans began in 1999, after which a pivotal study started in 2001. Of the 119 included patients, 88.1% had successful closure without adverse events, reintervention or significant residual shunt

at 12-month follow-up.[15] The major adverse event rate was 5.9%, including device embolization, inadequate device sizing requiring removal and nickel sensitivity. Most of the 27.7% minor adverse events were arrhythmias (5.0%), wire fractures (5.0%) and new onset migraine (4.2%). Residual leaks occurred in 2.6%. A subsequent FDA study reported success in 96.7% of patients with a 3.6% major adverse event rate at 5-year follow-up. As of now no cases of erosion had been reported. FDA approval of the HSO was received in 2006.

An HSO successor called Gore Septal Occluder (GSO), and more recently the Gore Cardioform Septal Occluder, was CE marked in 2011. GSO served to improve delivery and fixation by replacing nitinol with platinum and adding a porous coating and a delivery handle.

The GORE HELEX Septal Occluder (GSO) is made up of an implantable prosthesis and a catheter delivery system. The device is composed of expanded polytetrafluoroethylene (ePTFE) patch material with a hydrophilic coat, supported by a nickel-titanium (nitinol) super-elastic wire framework. Once the device is fully deployed, it takes a double-disc shape that first bridges, and over time occludes the defect to stop the shunting of blood between the left and right atriums. Double-disc nominal diameters range from 15 mm to 35 mm when completely deployed. The delivery system consists of three coaxial components: a mandrel, a 9Fr delivery catheter and a 6Fr control catheter. The control catheter has a retrieval cord to reposition and retrieve the device. The GORE HELEX Septal Occluder covers the defect and adjacent tissue with the ePTFE patch which is supported by the nitinol wire frame. Immediately after deployment, it remains in position across the defect with the help of the tension created by the wire frame and the blood pressure, which pushes the ePTFE patch against the septum. The PTFE patch is microporous and will become attached to the atrial septum by cellular penetration through the membrane micropores. Over time, the process of tissue attachment to the ePTFE patch will maintain the occluder in position and achieve a permanent defect closure.

The device is not recommended for larger defects (more than 18 mm), septal aneurysm, complex defects, septal thickness greater than 8 mm and multiple defects. The first experiences in children and adults supported compatibility with defects which were smaller than 18 mm.

OCCLUTECH FIGULLA FLEX OCCLUDER

The Occlutech Figulla ASD Occluder (FSO) device initially designed to close patent foramen ovales (PFOs) (Krizanic et al. 2008) is a double-disc system, similar to the ASO, with different structural modifications that make it quite attractive. This device is made of a nitinol wire mesh to create a smooth and flexible outer layer using a unique braiding technique so that the amount of metal is reduced by 50%. In addition the left atrial hub is removed. The two retention discs are connected with a central 4-mm waist, and the size of the device is determined by the diameter of the waist. The left atrial disc of the device is usually 12–16 mm larger than the waist and the right atrial disc is 8–11 mm larger. Polyester patches are sewn within both discs and the waist to improve thrombogenicity and to increase the occlusion rate of the defect. Compared with the ASO, the Figulla Flex Occluder has a reduced amount of material, with no hub on the left disc, so as to reduce the trauma risk and clot formation. The connecting system from the right disc to the distal tip of the delivery cable has evolved from a micro screw initially, as in the ASO, to a hub which is attached to the loader by two lateral hooks. With this latter connection, the double disc can be angled some 50 degrees without tension on the system. All these modifications have increased the flexibility of the device. The FSO is available in different sizes, ranging from 4 mm to 40 mm. Follow-up studies show almost no residual shunt in patients with ASD closure and one residual shunt in a patient whose PFO was closed.

Both FSO and ASO handle very well and can be recaptured or redeployed easily within the sheath, allowing appropriate repositioning, if necessary. However, the FSO is characterized by a reduction of material compared with the ASO. The absence of the distal hub on the left disc may be of benefit, in terms of reducing the risk of trauma, clot formation and subsequent systemic embolization. One of the main differences of the FSOs, compared to the ASOs, is the lack of the left-sided hub, which results in a softer left-sided disc despite comparable wire thickness. This creates a typical ball-shape appearance during deployment and results in less impingement on the surrounding structures.

Three generations of OFSOs have been released so far. These are available in different sizes, which range from as small as 4 mm to 40 mm in size. All the devices have CE approval. The first generation (Occlutech Septal Occluder N, OSO) had no left atrial hub, was credited CE mark in the year 2007 and was used with good results. The second generation (Flex Occluder) had a better delivery system that allowed tilt angle of 45 degrees, had a new ball-shaped connector design and achieved CE mark in 2009. The system allows septal alignment without any stress or tension on the septum, and thereby has improved flexibility during implantation. In the third-generation device (Flex II Occluder), the delivery system was changed to a bioptome-like delivery system, allowing a full circular movement, and less metal in the centre of the device provides better flexibility and a smaller delivery sheath requirement. All of these devices have a lower profile on the left atrial aspect/disc, with minimal impingement of the aortic vessel walls if placed adjacent to it. During deployment, the left atrial side develops in a round, ball-like shape, unlike the flat profile of other devices which possess a double-sided hub. This prevents the prolapse of the left-sided disc during the implantation process, especially in large ASDs or in those defects without or minimal aortic rim.

The IRFACODE project

In 1315 patients of all age groups (female 66.9%), successful (98%), ASD closure was performed (mean age 28.9 years, weight 52 kg, height 148.6 cm). Of all the defects, 47.9% had no or deficient aortic rim; in 11.9%, there was more than one defect; septum aneurysm was seen in 21.5%; and the mean implanted device size was 20.5 mm. Immediate closure was achieved in 78.6%, at discharge in 83.1%, and 96.4% and 97.3% at 6 and 12 months follow-up, respectively. During a mean follow-up of 2.7 years (in total 3597 patient years), significant complications were minimal with secondary device embolization in five and AV-blocks in three patients. No erosion or death was reported.

LIFETECH CERA ADS OCCULDER AND CERA FLEX

Cera ASD occluder (CSO) serves as an alternative to ASD due to high cost and unavailability in developing countries. The CeraFlex closure system is a percutaneous, transcatheter pre-loaded device developed by Lifetech Scientific for the interventional closure of ASD, MF-ASD, PDA and PFO.[17] The new, innovative CeraFlex pre-loaded occluder device is easy and convenient to use. With a maximum range of pivot of 360 degrees, the CeraFlex occluder allows for accurate positioning during the procedure. The new CeraFlex occluder, without a left-disc distal hub, is designed to minimize thrombotic complications. The new CeraFlex closure system series includes CeraFlex ASD, MF-ASD, PFO and PDA occluders as well as the SteerEase delivery device, and it is now more convenient and more user friendly. The state-of-the-art design and proprietary titanium nitride coating technology accelerate endothelialization, and prevent 93% of nickel release when compared with traditional uncoated occluders. All nitinol structures are plated with titanium nitride (TiN) to improve the biocompatibility. The CeraFlex occluders must be used in conjunction with the SteerEase delivery system. The delivery system contains a coil-reinforced sheath, a dilator and a haemostatic valve. And the CeraFlex delivery system includes an occluder, a loader, a haemostatic valve, a cable and a cable handle. The ceramic covering is designed to potentially reduce risk of thrombus formation and to cause fewer nickel ions to elute; and it has a TiN coating to enhance endothelialization.

A feasibility and safety study comparing CSO with ASO showed similar safety end points with lower cost. Also ASD >40 mm also can be closed like ASO devices.[17]

A more recent device CeraFlex differs mainly by an improved delivery system which provides 360-degree rotation at the tip to improve device positioning. The device received the CE mark in 2011. This was the first of Chinese brand marketed in Europe. Its feasibility and safety have been tested in clinical trials.

CARDIA ATRIA SEPTAL AND ULTRACEPT

Cradia Inc. developed several generations of occluder devices for PFOs and later for ASDs. The later generation devices were Atriasept I/II and Ultrasept I/II.[18] All generations had low-profile nitinol frames to minimize the device frame and enhance flexibility and had polyvinyl alcohol coating to reduce thrombus formation. Atriasept I had a squared disc with circular wires. There were reports of device perforation and atrial/aortic erosions. Atriasept II was improved using around disc but erosions were reported. The latest Cardia Ultrasept device, the seventh generation, has a polyvinyl alcohol (PVA) coating on its flower-like rounded discs. The device sizes range from 6 mm to 38 mm and corresponding 9-F to 11-F delivery sheath. It received CE marking in 2011. Device coating perforation is a major concern for this type of device.

SOLYSAFE SEPTAL OCLUDER

The Solysafe Septal Occluder (Swissimplant, Solothurn, Switzerland) was a self-centring device consisting of two polyester patches and eight wires made of cobalt alloy with two wire holders on each end. The wires were arranged in helical form and both ends were joined together by a snap-lock mechanism. A flat double-disc device was arranged as a flower shape. Device implantation required coaxial catheters which held the distal and proximal wire holders by a screwing mechanism, and the device would deploy by pulling the outer catheter and pushing the inner one. A presumed advantage was that a 10-F delivery sheath was needed only for femoral device introduction, since implantation was possible using the guidewire alone. Also, defect sizes up to 21 mm could be closed by either of three available device sizes. CE marking was received for these three sizes in 2007 and for two larger sizes in 2009. The Solysafe was discontinued in view of wire fractures and device fragmentation.

AMPLATZER SEPTAL OCCLUDER (ASD)

AGA Medical Corporation produces two types of ASD closure devices, namely the Amplatzer Septal Occluder (ASO) and the Cribriform Occluder. In 1997 the double-disc Amplazter Septal Occluder was developed with self-expanding and self-centring capabilities; the design served to reduce residual shunting and reduced incidence of frame fractures.[10] The device consisted of two discs, a larger left-side one and a smaller right-side disc connected by a nitinol waist between the two. The device required 6-F to 7-F sheaths for deployment. ASO is made from 004" to 007" nitinol wire with shape memory and with Dacron polyester patches sewn into each disc. The discs are connected by a 4-mm-long waist which sits within the defect.

The device is deployed in the left atrium, and after ensuring that the device does not impinge on nearby structures, the waist and right-side disc will be delivered. The device is self-centring and retractable into delivery sheath for repositioning if needed. Successful implantation was done in 96% of attempts with no major complications. Initial human experience by Hizaji et al. has shown promising results. The immediate closure rate demonstrated by transesophageal echocardiography and angiography was 17/30 patients (57%). However, within 24 hours of the procedure, the rate of complete closure increased to 24/30 (80%), and only 2/30 patients had moderate residual shunt. Furthermore, at 1-month follow-up, the closure rates had increased to 29/30 (97%). So far, no other device has achieved such a high complete closure rate. Some patients with residual shunt had undergone spontaneous closure or decrease in the degree of shunt in time, similar to patients with other devices. The unique design features (in particular, the connecting waist of this device, which in essence covers the defect), contribute to the immediate closure seen in the majority of the patients. IMPACT Registry and multicentre MAGIC study reported negligible complication rates.[9] ASO device embolization was the most frequent adverse event, followed by cardiac perforations which were reported in the range of 0.28%. Compared to occluders like CardioSEAL and STARFlex, the ASO's rate of thrombus formation is also very low. ASO is currently the most commonly used ASD closure device due to its straightforward deployment technique and easy retrievability and its ability to reposition at any time. FDA approval was obtained in 2001.[13] Despite its widespread use, device erosion both early and late is great cause for concern. Long-term surveillance is required.

AMPLATZER CRIBRIFORM DEVICE

The Amplatzer Cribriform device is used for closure of fenestrated ASDs. It has been fabricated in the same way as the ASO device. It consists of two equal-sized discs connected by a thin waist. The implantation technique is similar to that of the ASO device. The delivery sheath is positioned in middle fenestration and the disc should cover most peripheral fenestrations for effective closure. The device has shown satisfactory clinical outcomes.

COCOON ASD OCCLUDER (VASCULAR CONCEPTS, THAILAND)

The Cocoon Septal Occluder is made up from nitinol wires which are covered with platinum. The device is a self-expandable, double-disc device connected by a waist at the centre of the two discs. The discs are filled with polypropylene fabric to assist in thrombogenicity. Platinum provides superior bio-compatible properties compared with nitinol. It also prevents the corrosion of nitinol wire frameworks in long-term implants. Platinum also provides radio opacity, which assists in easy positioning. A preliminary European multicentre trial using Cocoon Septal Occluder was done in 92 patients. The device is an improved new-generation double-disc design made of nitinol wire mesh coated with platinum using Nano Fusion Technology. The discs are connected by a waist which actually covers the defect and is available in diameters ranging from 6 mm to 40 mm in size with 2-mm increments. In this study, complete closure of the defect immediately and at 1-month follow-up was observed in all 92 patients. No device-related complications were observed during the short-term follow-up of this study.

NIT-OCCLUDE ASD-R (NOASD-R)

NOASD-R is a device similar to the existing ones in terms of design. It is a double-disc self-expandable and self-centring device. Similar to the ASO, it is a one-piece nitinol frame without a hub on either side to minimize thrombosis and with polyester membrane sewn onto both discs to prevent device erosion and to enhance endothelialization. The devices range from 8 mm to 30 mm and are loaded on a 8–14-F sheath. At a multicentre trial in 2014, device erosions and device-induced complete heart block were noted during follow-up. CE approval was obtained for the device in 2012.

BIORESORBABLE SEPTAL OCCLUDER DEVICES

BioSTAR and BioTREK

The STARFlex device that was discontinued was later upgraded to BioSTAR by substituting polyester for porcine type I along with heparin coating.[19] The bioengineered collagen provides 90% of the structure, which starts absorbing by 30 days and is fully replaced by host tissue at about 2 years. The safety and efficacy of this device was tested in the BioSTAR evaluation study (BEST).[20] Closure rates of 92% to 96% were observed in the study. Concerns were raised in cases of larger defects, including the need for larger sheaths and longer procedural time. Dislocation of residual framework leading to aortic root perforation and/or late device embolization is a concern.

The BioSTAR device represents a landmark in the development of septal occluders. Its potential benefits include decreased long-term thrombogenicity, decreased inflammatory response, preserved transseptal access and reduced arrhythmogenicity and erosion potential. The lifespan and chronic mechanical stress upon the device are less important, since the implant is replaced by fibrous endothelialized tissue. One potential concern is resorption of the collagen matrix, prior to the overgrowth of endocardial tissue over the device, leading to a recurrent defect and shunt across the device. The device was tested in paediatric population by Benson et al., and testing found that acute and 6-month follow-up closure rates for the BioSTAR were 90% and 100% vs. 100% and 100% closure with the ASO implants.[14] There was a statistically significant difference in the median procedure time (52 minutes; BioSTAR: 39.5 minutes; ASO device: $P < 0.05$), with fluoroscopy times slightly longer for the BioSTAR group (6.7 minutes vs. 6.1 minutes, $P < 0.05$). There were no significant complications in either group.

BioTREK was a sequel to BioSTAR which would completely resorb without a metal framework.

It had good visibility on echocardiography and fluoroscopically, could be repositioned and was retrievable. Despite initial promising results, both occluders have been discontinued.

IMMEDIATE-RELEASE PATCH

Sideris et al. developed the innovative concept of wireless absorbable percutaneous closure devices, presenting the detachable balloon device and transcatheter patch. The older version required 48 hours of immobilization before deployment. The immediate-release patch (IRP) (Figure 7.2) is the recent version consisting of a porcine polyurethane sleeve patch with a surgical adhesive that allows immediate release and attachment.[21] The device can be deployed on the left atrial side by inflating a compliant balloon. It uses bioabsorbable Vicryl thread for repositioning and nylon thread for retrieval if necessary. Vicryl thread was sutured to groin subcutaneously and nylon thread was cut off once device was stable after 12 hours. Despite its appealing innovation, issues such as complex implantation technique, unsuitability for large defects, embolization and residual shunts remain a concern. These devices are being developed for closure of sinus venosus ASD types also.

CARAG BIORESORBABLE SEPTAL OCCLUDER

The Carag Bioresorbable Septal Occluder (CBSO) (Figure 7.2) is a self-centring flat polyester double disc which is repositionable and retractable without any metal framework. It is completely

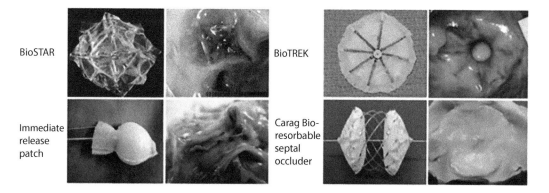

BioSTAR

BioTREK

Immediate release patch

Carag Bio-resorbable septal occluder

Figure 7.2 Bioabsorbable ASD closure devices. (Adapted from *Expert Review of Medical Devices*, 2016 Vol. 13, No. 6, 555–568.)

bioresorbable by 24 months with complete endothelialization and 100% success in preclinical studies. There have been no device-related adverse events reports so far. Similar to the IRP, three sizes are available for defects from 4 mm to 25 mm.

OTHER DEVICES

The Nit-Occlud PFO pfm closure device, the Sept Rx Intrapocket PFO Occluder, the Coherex Flatstent PFO device and radiofrequency technology by Sievert et al. are some of the devices attempted for ASD closure, but they are still in preclinical trials.

PFO-STAR DEVICE

The PFO-Star is a self-opening double umbrella developed for PFO closure. The device, also known as Atriasept II, is in its sixth generation. It is a self-centring device with nitinol frames with six arms and Ivalon attached to outside of frames.

PREMERE PFO CLOSURE SYSTEM

The Premere occluder designed by St. Jude Medical was designed for PFO occlusion. It has two cross-shaped nitinol arms with the left atrial side being uncovered and a right-side anchor covered on both sides with a knitted polyester membrane. It has been available since 2005 in some countries.

PFx CLOSURE SYSTEM

The PFx Closure System is a non-device system for PFO closure. It is a percutaneous system that employs monopolar radiofrequency energy to effect closure of PFO by welding the tissue between septum primum and secundum together. The catheter need not enter into left atrium, so no thrombus formation occurs. But due to low closure rates this technology was discontinued in 2009.

AMPLATZER PFO OCCLUDER

The Amplatzer Occluder is the only available device that has an FDA approval for PFO closure in the setting of cryptogenic stroke. It is composed of two nitinol woven discs with integral Dacron patches and a fixed short waist. The patches are designed to stimulate endothelialization. The device comes in multiple sizes with the right atrial disc being larger than the left. One exception is the 18-mm device, which has equal-sized bi-atrial discs.

TISSUE-ENGINEERED MEMBRANES

Many of the limitations of our current series of devices could be overcome with the development of autologous tissue-engineered membranes mounted on a biodegradable scaffold.[22] The result would be closure of a defect using one's own tissue with no foreign material left behind as the scaffold degrades. But it is still in its infancy and not in clinical use.

HEARTSTITCH

Heartstitch used a transcatheter suture system to close septal defects. The device was delivered into the left atrium and septum primum, was sutured to secundum and the catheter withdrawn. But due to technical difficulties the system went out of use.

The current FDA-approved and CE-approved devices have excellent success and closure rates, but each device has its strength and weakness. A timeline of various ASD devices is shown in Figure 7.3.[1] A double disc with a short waist proved to be a more robust device during initial days, but now ideal frame material and covering has been given importance even though an ideal material has not been found yet.

With 20 years' experience the ASO device stands test of time, and the design has been modelled for subsequent devices like the Occlutech and Lifetech occluders. Nonetheless, risk of cardiac erosion remains a concern. The Occlutech devices have flexible delivery systems, which suit patients with deficient rims. But due to reduced materials the risks of embolization and residual shunts have to be dealt with. Therefore, newer methods to produce wireless bioabsorbable devices are being tried to overcome shortcomings.

Even though bioabsorbable devices appear to be an appealing option because of absence of foreign materials and lack of wire-related complications, the potential for residual shunts and recurrent defects must be kept in mind. Until these challenges are overcome, current devices with their inherent strengths and weakness have to be pursued and

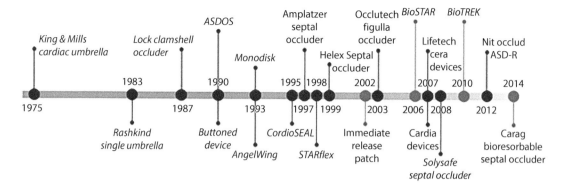

Figure 7.3 Timeline of ASD devices from 1975 to present. (Adapted from *Expert Review of Medical Devices*, 2016 Vol. 13, No. 6, 555–568.)

used accordingly for each specific group of defects. Long-term surveillance is essential for assessing efficacy against safety and thereby direct current clinical practice to optimization.

There is now increasing confidence in the safety and success of currently available percutaneous closure devices with which even complex defects such as deficient rims, septal aneurysms, multiple or large defects (>35 mm), and multiple fenestrations are being closed successfully. Even surgical closure indications for device embolization will be replaced by percutaneous repairs. The anticipated outcomes of new generation bioabsorbable ASD closure devices will determine the future course in ASD treatment, limiting the need for invasive surgical procedures. If successful, they are going to become the choice of device, making metallic devices an alternative in the future.

CONCLUSION

The range of ASD closure devices available in the market has made percutaneous closure of simple and complex atrial septal defects possible. Safety and feasibility studies have shown high levels of procedural success and recognizable features that predisposes to complications. The wide range of available sizes is being utilized for closing most of the defects, with a negligible number of cases requiring surgical intervention. The introduction of biodegradable technology and nickel-free product may minimize long-term sequelae. The continued development of ASD device technology, as well as long-term success with current devices, will ensure that percutaneous ASD closure is a preferred approach.

REFERENCES

1. Nassif M, Abdelghani M, Bouma BJ, et al. Historical developments of atrial septal defect closure devices: What we learn from the past. *Expert Rev. Med. Devices.* 2016; 13(6):555–568.
2. Alapati, S, Rao, PS. (2012). Historical aspects of transcatheter occlusion of atrial septal defects. Doi: 10.5772/38930.
3. Alexi-Meskishvili VV, Konstantinov IE. Surgery for atrial septal defect: From the first experiments to clinical practice. *Ann Thorac Surg.* 2003; 76:322–27.
4. King TD, Thompson SL, Steiner C, et al. Secundum atrial septal defect: Nonoperative closure during cardiac catheterization. *JAMA.* 1976; 235:2506–09.
5. Mills NL, King TD. Late follow-up of nonoperative closure of secundum atrial septal defects using the King-mills double-umbrella device. *Am J Cardiol.* 2003; 92:353–55.
6. Beekman RH, Rocchini AP, Snider AR. Transcatheter atrial septal defect closure: Preliminary experience with the Rashkind occlude device. *J Interv Cardiol.* 1989; 2(1):35–41.
7. Sievert H, Babic UU, Hausdorf G, et al. Transcatheter closure of atrial septal defect and patent foramen ovale with ASDOS device (a multi-institutional European trial). *Am J Cardiol.* 1998; 82(11):1405–13.
8. Pavcnik D, Wright KC, Wallace S. Monodisk: Device for percutaneous transcatheter closure of cardiac septal defects. *Cardiovasc Intervent Radiol.*1993; 16(5):308–12.

9. Everett AD, Jennings J, Sibinga E, et al. Community use of the Amplatzer atrial septal defect occluder: Results of the multicenter MAGIC atrial septal defect study. *Pediatr Cardiol.* 2009; 30(3): 240–47.

10. Fu YC, Hijazi ZM. The Amplatzer Septal Occluder, a transcatheter device for atrial septal defect closure. *Expert Rev Med Devices.* 2008; 5:25–31.

11. Magni G, Hijazi ZM, Pandian NG, et al. Two- and three-dimensional transesophageal echocardiography in patient selection and assessment of atrial septal defect closure by the new DAS-Angel Wings device: Initial clinical experience. *Circulation.* 1997; 96:1722–28.

12. Nugent AW, Britt A, Gauvreau K, et al. Device closure rates of simple atrial septal defects optimized by the STARFlex device. *J Am Coll Cardiol.* 2006; 48(3):538–544.

13. Rao PS, Berger F, Rey C, et al. Results of transvenous occlusion of secundum atrial septal defects with the fourth generation buttoned device: Comparison with first, second and third generation *devices. International Buttoned Device Trial group. J Am Coll Cardiol.* 2000; 36: 583–92.

14. Bennhagen RG, McLaughlin P, Benson LN. CardioSeal and STARFlex devices. In: Rao PS, Kern MJ, editors. *Catheter based devices for treatment of noncoronary cardiovascular disease in adults and children.* Philadelphia (PA): Lippincott, Williams & Wilkins; 2003. 61–69.

15. Moore J, Hegde S, El-Said H, et al. Transcatheter device closure of atrial septal defects: A safety review. *JACC Cardiovasc Interv.* 2013; 6:433–42.

16. Jones TK, Latson LA, Zahn E, et al. Results of the U.S. multicenter pivotal study of the HELEX Septal Occluder for percutaneous closure of secundum atrial septal defects. *J Am Coll Cardiol,* 2007; 49:2215–2221.

17. Kaya MG, Akpek M, Celebi A, et al. A multicentre, comparative study of Cera septal occluder versus Amplatzer Septal Occluder in transcatheter closure of secundum atrial septal defects. *EuroIntervention.* 2014; 10: 626–631.

18. Stolt VS, Chessa M, Aubry P, et al. Closure of ostium secundum atrial septum defect with the Atriasept occluder: Early European experience. *Catheter Cardiovasc Interv.* 2010; 75:1091–10.

19. Jux C, Bertram H, Wohlsein P, et al. Interventional atrial septal defect closure using a totally bioresorbable occluder matrix: Development and preclinical evaluation of the BioSTAR device. *J Am Coll Cardiol.* 2006; 48:161–69.

20. Morgan G, Lee KJ, Chaturvedi R, et al. A biodegradable device (BioSTAR) for atrial septal defect closure in children. *Catheter Cardiovasc Interv.* 2010; 76:241–45.

21. Zeinaloo A, Zanjani KS, Rastkar B, et al. Closure of interatrial defects by immediate-release patch. *Pediatr Cardiol.* 2012; 33:1253–58.

22. Sievert H. First human use and intermediate follow-up of a septal occluder with bioresorbable framework. EuroPCR 2015; Euro15AOP336, 2015; May 19; Paris.

8

Role of echocardiography in transcatheter device closure

A HANDA

Diagnosis of atrial septal defects (ASDs) is largely by echocardiography. Cardiac CT and MRI can give valuable information regarding quantification of shunt and haemodynamics. Echocardiography is used for imaging guidance during percutaneous transcatheter closure of ASDs and patent foramen ovales (PFOs). Real-time intraprocedural echocardiography TTE, TEE, 3D imaging or ICE provide vital information before, during and after deployment of the device.[1] Although each modality has its own advantages and disadvantages, echocardiographic augmentation of fluoroscopic imaging offers significant information in individual patient selection, device selection, procedural guidance, monitoring for complications and assessment of the results.

IMAGING MODALITIES IN TRANSCATHETER GUIDANCE

Transthoracic echocardiography, transesopahageal and intracardiac echo

Regardless of modality, baseline transthoracic echocardiography is essential in the monitoring of transcatheter procedure guidance and post-procedural complications. A list of all major complications of transcatheter closure and the appropriate imaging modality to assist with the diagnosis is provided in Table 8.1.

Transthoracic echocardiography is the baseline invasive imaging modality for percutaneous transcatheter closure and could be adequate for procedure guidance in smaller patients.[2] Its limitations include suboptimal imaging in larger patients and interference of the echocardiographic probe with fluoroscopy.[2] In addition, the implanted device creates artefacts, frequently precluding interrogation of the lower rim of the atrial septal tissue above the inferior vena cava (IVC). Transesophageal echocardiography provides detailed imaging findings during percutaneous transcatheter closure.

General anaesthesia can be used whenever TEE is performed to enhance patient comfort and improve imaging anatomy and better delineation of the intended structure for analysis. In addition to the anaesthetist, a dedicated echocardiographer is optional to perform the TEE during the closure procedure. In selected cases conscious sedation can be used rather than general anaesthesia.

Table 8.1 Acute and chronic complications of percutaneous transcatheter closure and role of echocardiography in diagnosis and treatment

Complication	Consequence	Acuity	Treatment	Role of echocardiography	Preferred echocardiographic modality
Cardiac perforation	Cardiac tamponade	Acute	Emergency surgery	Diagnostic	TTE, TEE or ICE
Device embolization	Embolization, valve obstruction	Acute or chronic	Percutaneous or surgical retrieval	Diagnosis, guidance of percutaneous retrieval	TTE, TEE or ICE for diagnosis; TEE or ICE for retrieval
Bleeding	Hypovolemia	Shock, death	Acute transfusion, surgical intervention	Excluding other diagnoses	TTE

Intracardiac echocardiography has emerged as an alternative imaging modality for transcatheter closure guidance. ICE imaging is comparable to TEE and more helpful for LA structures and the postero-inferior rim of the septum.[3] The ICE system requires additional logistics, especially 8-F to 11-F sheaths. If the patient weights more than 35 kg, then sheaths for both the device and the ICE system can be placed in the same femoral vein using two separate punctures several millimetres apart. In thinner patients, venous access for the ICE catheter should be obtained in the contralateral vein. Although separate echocardiographic expertise is helpful for providing assistance during the procedure, it is not always required as the interventionalist performing the septal closure can also manipulate the catheter. The procedure does not require general anaesthesia. Also shorter procedure and shorter fluoroscopy times are possible, and the cost is lower compared to TEE-guided percutaneous closure, where use of general anaesthesia is essential.[4]

Three-dimensional ICE has been introduced recently, and the preliminary results have started emerging from evaluating patients with structural heart disease. Three-dimensional TEE offers live real-time imaging of the septum, providing a comprehensive analysis of the defect and its relationship to the surrounding structures.[5] Direct visualization of the deployed device from both sides of interatrial septum augments the post-deployment assessment of the defect and efficacy

of the device closure and potential complications associated with the procedure.

INTRAPROCEDURAL GUIDANCE OF TRANSCATHETER INTERVENTIONS[6]

All patients undergoing percutaneous transcatheter closure of septal defects require pre-procedural echocardiographic imaging, with either TTE or TEE, to assess the septal anatomy and determine the suitability of an atrial defect for device closure.[2] This includes a detailed echocardiographic investigation of the entire IAS and surrounding structures using multiple sequential planes, as previously defined. The different type of ASD (ASD type, ASA, PFO), the number of defects adjacent to main defect (up to 13% of patients could have more than one defect), defect size, its location, morphology and the surrounding atrial septal tissue (rims) should be delineated (Table 8.1). Other associated abnormalities of the adjoining structures such as the pulmonary veins, IVC, SVC, coronary sinus, eustachian valve and AV valves should be evaluated. The septal defect and surrounding rims of atrial tissue should be carefully evaluated. Using TEE with the midesophageal four-chamber view (starting from 0" multiplane and moving in 15" multiplane increments), the inferior–anterior and superior–posterior rims can be defined (Figures 8.1–8.3). The anterior rim or the aortic rim of the atrial septal defect and the posterior rim are measured in the midesophageal

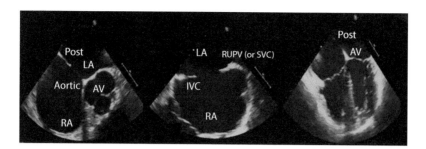

Figure 8.1 Images representing three (of five) views for assessment of ASD by TEE. Short-axis views are critical for the assessment of the aortic rim and device interaction with the aorta. Bicaval and long-axis views (not shown) are critical for the assessment of the relationship of the device with the roofs of the atrium. AV: atrioventricular valve rim; Post: posterior rim. (Adapted from ASE guidelines for echocardiographic assessment of ASD and PFO, August 2015.)

short-axis view (30"–45" multiplane and moving in 15" increments). The midesophageal bicaval view (110"–130") is used to visualize the superior as well as inferior rims. Imaging with 3D TEE allows for acquisition of similar sets of data but without the need for serial assessment in multiple stepwise

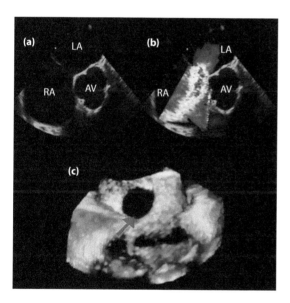

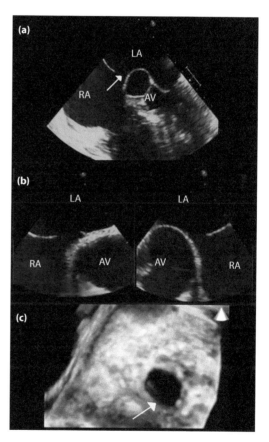

Figure 8.2 Three-dimensional TEE of medium-sized ostium secundum ASD with a mildly deficient aortic rim. Midesophageal aortic valve short-axis view demonstrates the ASD and the aortic rim deficiency (a). Identical view demonstrating the left-to-right shunting by colour Doppler flow (b). Zoom mode of ASD en face from RA perspective (c). Red arrow specifies ASD. AV: aortic valve. (Adapted from ASE guidelines for echocardiographic assessment of ASD and PFO, August 2015.)

Figure 8.3 Three-dimensional TEE of medium-sized ostium secundum ASD with a deficient aortic rim. Modified midesophageal four-chamber view (a). Biplane image demonstrating multiple areas of deficiency (b). Zoom mode of ASD en face from LA perspective (c). Yellow arrow specifies a deficient rim; yellow arrow, ASD. AV: aortic valve. (Adapted from ASE guidelines for echocardiographic assessment of ASD and PFO, August 2015.)

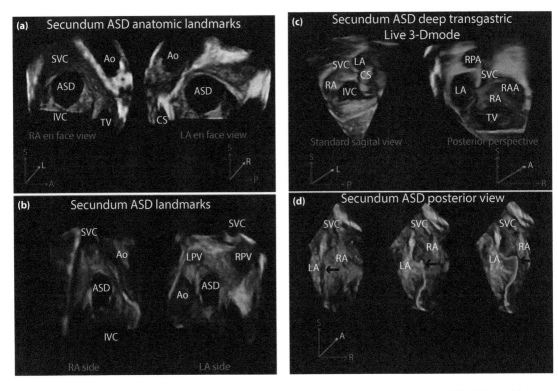

Figure 8.4 Representative views and anatomic landmarks in an ostium secundum ASD. RA and LA en face views (a and b). Transgastric sagittal bicaval view in live 3D mode from the standard perspective (c). Posterior views demonstrating the variable alignment between the septum primum and secundum over the entire cardiac cycle (d). Alignment between the septum secundum and septum primum (arrow) components (left). Mild malalignment (middle) and more malalignment (right) present between the septal components. As the malalignment tends to increase, the size of the interatrial communication (asterisk) increases. In the orientation icon, blue designates the y plane, red, the x plane, and green, the z plane. (Adapted from ASE guidelines for echocardiographic assessment of ASD and PFO, August 2015.)

views (Figures 8.4 and 8.5). Also transgastric imaging could be required to visualize the inferior rim of an ASD in some cases and can be used to define the relationship of the inferior aspects of the device and the IAS.[4]

ICE GUIDANCE OF ASD DEVICE CLOSURE

When using ICE, a full assessment of the defect and surrounding tissue rims should be performed. The probe is positioned such that the tricuspid valve is first identified. From this position, a posterior deflection of the knob with a slight rightward rotation of the right–left knob will obtain the septal view.[7] Advancing the catheter cephalad produces the bicaval view, from which the superior and inferior rims and the defect diameter are measured (Figure 8.6a). Rotation of the handle clockwise until the transducer is near the tricuspid valve, followed by a leftward rotation of the right–left knob until the AoV appears, creates a view similar to the TEE short-axis plane, with the difference being the near field with ICE is the RA versus that with TEE showing the LA (Figure 8.6b). From this view, the diameter of the defect and the aortic and posterior rims can be measured. A complete 'neutral' sweep should be performed, starting and ending at the 'home view' to be performed.[8] This will effectively exclude sinus venosus SVC-type ASDs, evaluate any AV valve regurgitation and provide a comprehensive over view of entire atrial septum. This should be performed before device placement and again after to evaluate for mitral regurgitation

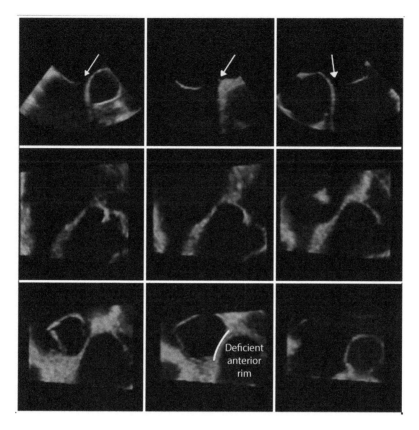

Figure 8.5 Three-dimensional TEE facilitates en face assessment of ASD shape and size and can characterize the degree of deficiency of the rims. The aortic rim is shown to be deficient in the bottom centre image slice. (Adapted from ASE guidelines for echocardiographic assessment of ASD and PFO, August 2015.)

and tricuspid regurgitation. A full sweep both of the bicaval and AoV views usually can be done with the catheter having a posterior tilt and pointing directly anterior in the RA.[8]

The initial echocardiographic assessment should include measurement of the defect diameter in the orthogonal planes, overall septal length and defect rims (retro-aortic, inferior–IVC and posterior–pulmonary vein). If multiple defects are present, each should be characterized and the distance separating them measured. In addition to echocardiographic data, a thorough right and left heart hemodynamic assessment is performed to determine the physiologic significance of the defect and exclude any anatomic or physiologic contraindications to septal closure. Right upper pulmonary venous angiography (35″ left anterior oblique with 35″ cranial angulation) can be performed to profile the atrial septum and serve as a fluoroscopic road map during device deployment.[2]

Balloon sizing of the defect with fluoroscopic and echocardiographic imaging is recommended for all ASD device closure cases; however, some operators might choose not to perform balloon sizing owing to the dimensions of the defect. The stop-flow technique involves placement of a sizing balloon across the interatrial defect.[2] During imaging with colour Doppler, slow inflation of the balloon is performed until colour flow across the defect has completely ceased (Figure 8.7a). The diameter of the balloon within the atrial defect is measured in several imaging planes at the point at which the flow across the defect is eliminated. It is also essential to interrogate the septum during balloon occlusion of the defect in two orthogonal views (short axis and bicaval) to identify or exclude the presence of additional defects. Once sizing has been completed, the ICE catheter is moved back to the long axis to monitor the various steps of closure[9] (Figure 8.7).

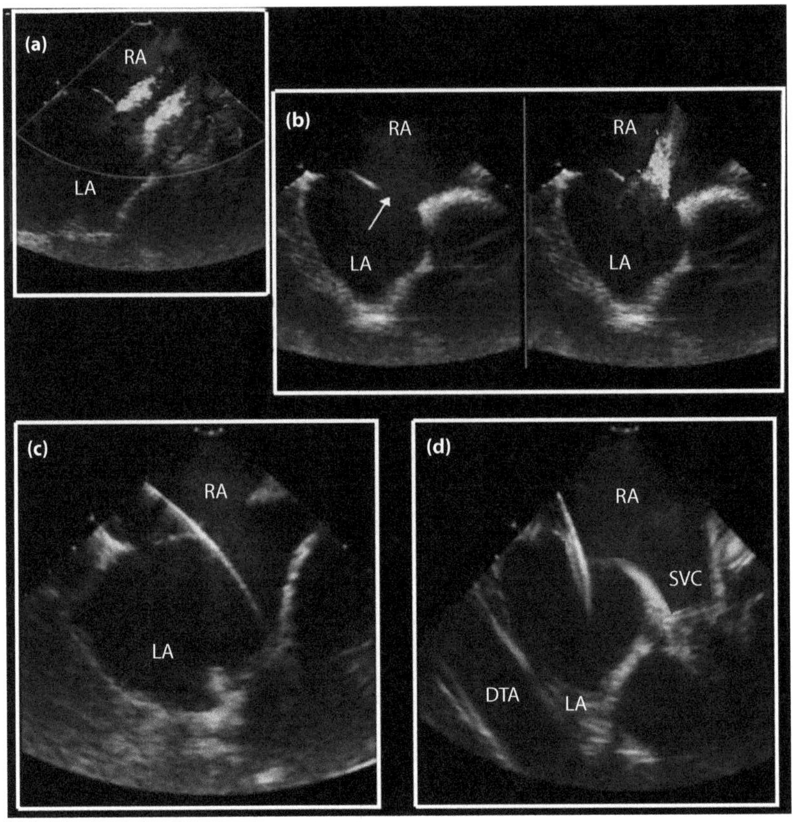

Figure 8.6 Intracardiac echocardiographically guided ASD closure of ostium secundum defect. Pre-procedure images demonstrating the ostium secundum ASD (a and b). Yellow arrow specifies the ASD. Passage of guidewire into the LSPV (c). Passage of guide catheter into LA (d). DTA: descending thoracic aorta. LSPV: left superior pulmonary vein. (Adapted from ASE guidelines for echocardiographic assessment of ASD and PFO, August 2015.)

IMAGING THE IAS IMMEDIATELY AFTER THE PROCEDURE

Echocardiographic guidance during deployment of ASD occlusion devices is used to monitor all stages of device delivery. The most useful views with TEE are the four-chamber and short-axis views. With ICE, the bicaval view gives a panoramic image of the entire left atrium (Figure 8.6). For the ASO, a device between the stop-flow diameter and up to 2 mm greater than the measured size is selected. The delivery system is introduced through the venous sheath and advanced into the left upper pulmonary vein (Figures 8.6 and 8.7). The wire and the dilator (both) are slowly withdrawn, taking care to eliminate the possibility of air embolism. The device is loaded and advanced to the tip of the sheath. The delivery sheath is then repositioned into the body of the LA from the pulmonary vein. The interventionalist fixes the cable and retracts the sheath, thus deploying the LA disc (Figure 8.7b). It is important to understand that echocardiography shows to the operator that the LA disc is remote from the pulmonary veins or LA appendage. Once the left disc is within a few millimetres from the septum, the connecting waist is deployed partially in the LA with continuous traction towards the defect (Figure 8.7c). The aim is to 'stent' the defect with the waist. Next, with continuous traction towards the RA, the RA disc is deployed (Figure 8.7 d & e). Once the entire disc is away from the tip of the sheath, the delivery cable is advanced towards the septum to bring the two discs of the device into approximation (Figure 8.7e).

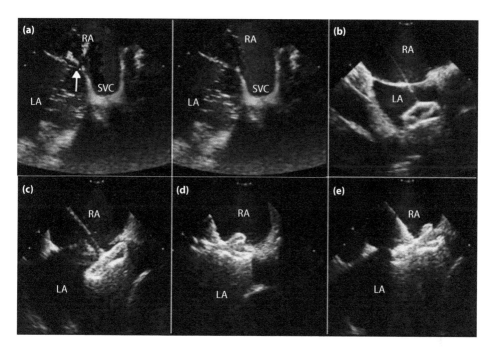

Figure 8.7 ICE-guided ASD closure of ostium secundum type of defect. Balloon sizing of the defect with and without colour Doppler (a). Arrow specifies a small degree of trivial flow around the balloon. Left atrial disc opens and is being withdrawn towards the interatrial septum (b). Withdrawal of the LA disc towards the IAS (c). Both discs are opened, and the position is checked to ensure the septum is 'sandwiched' between the discs (d and e). (Adapted from ASE guidelines for echocardiographic assessment of ASD and PFO, August 2015.)

In the case of Helex Septal Occluder (W.L. Gore), the ratio of the device to defect diameter should always be more than 2:1, but the diameter of the device should be not be more than 90% of the total septal length. Under fluoroscopic and echocardiographic (TTE) visualization, the catheter tip of the Helex delivery system (W.L. Gore) is advanced across the ASD until the radiopaque marker is positioned within the LA. The left atrial occluder disc is formed in the body of the LA. The interventionalist relies primarily on fluoroscopic imaging for this manoeuvre. If TEE is used, it might be beneficial to pull the probe back out of the fluoroscopic image. Once the LA disc is formed, echocardiographic imaging TTE or TEE is used to guide the positioning of the device against the left side aspect of the septum.[6] The LA disc is fixed against the septal tissue while the delivery catheter is withdrawn into the RA and by that movement the RA disc is formed. Echocardiographic assessment is repeated to confirm that both the discs appear planar and apposed to the septum with septal tissue between the discs. For both the Helex device and the ASO, a complete assessment of the device, septal anatomy and surrounding structures is performed before release of the device. Two orthogonal views are essential to verify that the LA and RA discs are both located in the correct chamber respectively. Colour Doppler is performed to exclude residual flow at the device margins, the presence of which suggests inappropriate device size or position (Figure 8.8). Proper imaging is performed to identify the entrapment of atrial septal tissue between both device discs. The aortic rim is easily seen, and extreme care must be taken to identify the presence of both important posterior as well as inferior tissue. Obstruction of pulmonary veins, coronary sinus and AV valve function, as well as deformation of the aortic root are carefully assessed and excluded before release. Possible device impingement on adjoining structures, especially the aorta, should be assessed. After the device has been deployed, assessment with TTE or TEE should be performed again. The role of three-dimensional

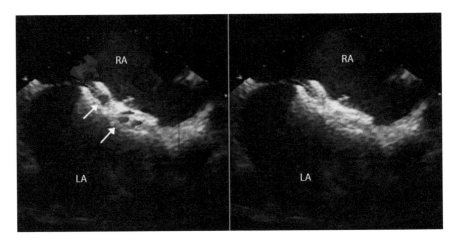

Figure 8.8 ICE-guided closure of ostium secundum ASD defect. The final device position (after release from guiding cable) demonstrates normal small residual leak (arrows) through the device. (Adapted from ASE guidelines for echocardiographic assessment of ASD and PFO, August 2015.)

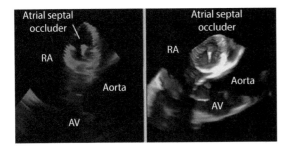

Figure 8.9 Three-dimensional ICE demonstrating the relationship of the atrial septal occluder to the aorta in 2D (left) and 3D (right) imaging modes. ASO: atrial septal occluder. (Adapted from ASE guidelines for echocardiographic assessment of ASD and PFO, August 2015.)

ICE has not yet been clearly defined, but it offers potential for additional anatomic delineation at the transcatheter closure[10] (Figure 8.9).

FOLLOW-UP

A transthoracic echocardiography study should be performed before discharge and repeated after a week when the Amplatzer device is used. Care should be given to the device position, any residual shunt, evidence of device erosion or deformation of the surrounding structures. The presence of a pericardial effusion could be an indication of device erosion. A 12-lead electrocardiography should also be performed because rare cases of heart block have been reported with large devices. Higher incidence of atrial arrhythmias and conduction abnormalities early after device closure has been reported. Follow-up evaluations, preferably TTE and selected case TEE, should be performed at 1, 6 and 12 months after the procedure, with a further evaluation every 1–2 years. For the Helex Septal Device (W.L. Gore), attention should also be given to the stability of the device, as lack of device stability could indicate wire or frame damage. In instances where device stability is an issue, fluoroscopic examination is recommended to identify and assess wire frame fractures. The RV size will improve rapidly in the first month after correction of the left-to-right shunt; however, prolonged RV dilation might improve more slowly and also might not normalize completely.

REFERENCES

1. Vaidyanathan B, Simpson JM, Kumar RK. Transesophageal echocardiography for device closure of atrial septal defects: Case selection, planning, and procedural guidance. *JACC Cardiovasc Imaging.* 2009; 2: 238–42.
2. Takaya Y, Akagi T, Nakagawa K, Ito H. Integrated 3D echo-x-ray navigation guided transcatheter closure of complex multiple atrial septal defects. *JACC Cardiovasc Interv.* 2016; 9(12):e111–12.

3. Vigna C, Marchese N, Zanchetta M, et al. Echocardiographic guidance of percutaneous patent foramen ovale closure: Head-to-head comparison of transesophageal versus rotational intracardiac echocardiography. *Echocardiography* 2012; 29:1103–10.

4. Roberson DA, Cui W, Patel D, et al. Three dimensional transesophageal echocardiography of atrial septal defect: A qualitative and quantitative anatomic study. *J Am Soc Echocardiogr.* 2011; 24:600–10.

5. Abdel-Massih T, Dulac Y, Taktak A, et al. Assessment of atrial septal defect size with 3D-transesophageal echocardiography: Comparison with balloon method. *Echocardiography* 2005; 22:121–7.

6. Bartel T, Müller S. Device closure of interatrial communications: Peri-interventional assessment. *Eur Heart J Cardiovasc Imaging* 2013; 14:618–24.

7. Kavvouras C, Vavuranakis M, Vaina S, et al. Intarcardiac echocardiography for percutaneous patent foramen ovale and atrial septal defect occlusion. *Herz.* 2019; 44(5):445–49.

9. Balzer D. Intracardiac echocardiographic atrial septal defect closure. *Methodist Debakey Cardiovasc J.* 2014; 10(2):88–92.

8. Hernández F, García-Tejada J, Velázquez M, Albarrán A, Andreu J, Tascón J. Intracardiac echocardiography and closure of atrial septal defects. *Rev Esp Cardiol.* 2008; 61(5):465–70.

10. Medford BA, Taggart NW, Cabalka AK. Intracardiac echocardiography during atrial septal defect and patent foramen ovale device closure in pediatric and adolescent patients. *J Am Soc Echocardiogr.* 2014: 27(9):984–990.

9

Transcatheter closure techniques

A A PILLAI, A HANDA

STANDARD TRANSCATHETER CLOSURE TECHNIQUE

All patients are scrutinized for the indication of atrial septal defect (ASD) closure. Preferably all patients should have a pre-procedure TTE and TEE. TEE imaging in small or paediatric patients is usually performed during the procedure. TEE imaging of all complex defects is usually done with 120 degrees sweeping in addition to the standard imaging angles at 0, 45 and 90 degrees. The size of the defect, shape of the defect, number of defects and location with regard to mitral valve and aortic valve are noted. Each of the important rims is measured and documented. Malalignment and aneurysm should also be noted.

Patients selected for transcatheter closure are given a loading dose of an antiplatelet agent (aspirin 300 mg or 4 mg/kg) one day before the procedure. Local anaesthesia, mild sedation and TTE during procedure are standard for all adult patients. General anaesthesia is used for all paediatric patients, and TEE can be used as per institutional protocol in all/selective cases. Femoral venous access is commonly used for transcatheter closure, while femoral arterial access is used for invasive pressure monitoring during the procedure. Anticoagulation should be achieved using 100 U/kg unfractionated heparin, with activated clotting time (ACT) maintained between 250 and 300 seconds throughout the procedure. Femoral venous access is then used for crossing the defect using a 5F/6F Cournard or multipurpose catheter with 0.035" hydrophilic guide wire. After crossing the defect the Cournard catheter is parked in left or right upper pulmonary vein. This catheter is then exchanged for 0.038" super stiff wire for supporting the long device-delivery sheath. The respective device is then loaded and delivered.[1]

MODIFIED TECHNIQUES FOR COMPLEX ASD CLOSURES

The ASD closure with standard deployment technique fails many patients, but modified techniques can be used. In some patients, with very large devices/floppy rims, one can straight away attempt the modified techniques.[2]

BALLOON SIZING OF DEFECTS

ASD sizing balloon with stop-flow technique can be used upon the operator's discretion. In cases where there is a malalignment defect, defects with septal aneurysm and where there is suboptimal sizing with TEE, balloon sizing with a stop-flow echo technique and fluoroscopic measurement can be an extremely useful method.

PULMONARY VEIN DEPLOYMENT TECHNIQUE

In this method, the left atrial disc is completely deployed in the pulmonary vein; keeping the disc in pulmonary vein, the whole device is stretched out to open the right atrial disc. Momentary release of the left atrial disc is done when the right atrial disc fans out to catch the two sides of the septum. This technique can be attempted in left upper, right upper and sometimes in left lower pulmonary vein.

LEFT ATRIAL ROOF DEPLOYMENT METHOD

This uses the same principle as in pulmonary vein deployment, but the left disc is opened against the left atrial roof.

MODIFIED/CUT SHEATH APPROACH

Here the operator cuts the sheath tip in an oblique fashion to allow for asymmetric expansion of the left atrial disc to catch the rims of the defect, followed by the asymmetric deployment of the right atrial disc. This method is used in cases of malaligned septum.

DILATOR/CATHETER-ASSISTED METHOD

With the help of a contralateral venous access, a long dilator/diagnostic catheter–wire assembly is kept across the defect to support the device delivery. This method can be used in cases with deficient posterior/aortic rims, where the device tends to slip back into right atrium in the conventional approach.

BALLOON-ASSISTED TECHNIQUE (BAT)

Here again with the help of a contralateral venous sheath, a highly compliant sizing balloon is used to occlude the defect fully or partially for supporting the device delivery. The device is then delivered from either the left upper or right upper pulmonary vein, and the balloon over the wire is placed on the contra lateral side. With the inflated balloon in situ across the defect, the LA disc is deployed and then the assembly pulled back to the septum. The balloon supports and prevents prolapse of the LA disc into the RA and then allows the delivery of the RA disc outside of the sheath. Then, after checking the discs on their respective sides of the septum by TEE, the operator deflates the balloon slowly, allowing the discs to expand and stent the septum, followed by careful, slow and steady withdrawal of the balloon. This method is useful in deployment of devices larger than 35 mm and with deficient/floppy margins.[3]

OUR EXPERIENCE WITH MODIFIED TECHNIQUES

We recently analyzed our data on 373 patients who had larger ASD measuring ≥30 mm (unpublished data). Three parameters proved statistically significant in procedural outcomes: very large defect size measuring ≥40 mm, deficient posterior margin and deficient inferior vena caval margin. We had very few cases of deficient superior vena caval and deficient coronary sinus margins (<1%).[4]

In our experience, spanning more than three decades with transesophageal echocardiographic imaging of atrial septal defects, most of the anatomic complexities are seen more common with larger defects like the ones in this study. Nearly 80% patients had a deficient posterior rim, inferior caval rim or septal malalignment. This made the success of conventional techniques very low (8%) in this series. The larger mean defect size of 35.3 mm with 22% patients having defects ≥40 mm was another feature in this group, which could have played a role in lowering the success of conventional techniques. Absent retro aortic margin was the most common anatomic variation reported in the literature, and we had about 42% patients with this deficiency. This anomaly was not a factor for procedural failure in our series. Presence of septal aneurysm or multiple defects did not show an outcome difference either. However, the aneurysm was found to result in significant discrepancy in the measurement of defect size. We found a mean size difference of 2.3 mm ± 1.5 mm in patients with and without septal aneurysm between transesophageal echocardiogram and the balloon stop-flow technique.

Septal malalignment is a rarely reported situation in transcatheter closure. We found that the lack of alignment of septum primum and secundum in the form of L or S shape interferes with proper disc alignment. For a successful closure with a double umbrella device, the expanded left atrial disc has to fall in line with the septal plane so that the right atrial disc can be released to about the right side of the septum. The left atrial disc should be held against the defect on the left atrial side for the waist to expand across the defect and the subsequent expansion of the right disc. A balloon-assisted technique was helpful in cases with nonlinear septal planes. With the modified techniques, the success rate was 78%. We feel that the combination of absent retro aortic margin with malalignment is unfavourable as it eventually precludes any sort of left atrial disc alignment against the septum, causing it to tilt tangentially across the defect; balloon assistance helps in this type of anomaly.

Posterior and inferior vena caval margins are often regarded as crucial for holding the device. Complete absence of entire posterior and inferior caval margins essentially rules out a device intervention in our practice. But if either of them was adequate, the case was attempted. The device can be successfully placed if the lower half of the semicircular, or C-shaped, ridge (comprising the posterior margin above and inferior vena caval margin below) is strong. Absent or floppy posterior margin poses difficulty in device alignment. Combined absence of diametrically opposite anterior and posterior septal margins is a challenge to deploy the device as most often the left disc tilts down. We find the balloon-assisted technique useful in this situation as it temporarily holds the left disc while the waist is deployed followed by right disc. In our experience, this works very well as the inflated balloon holds onto the whole system until the whole device is delivered, and device tends to be stable in such cases when the inferior half of the 'C' or the inferior caval margin is good and strong to support the device. However, if this margin is not good, then the device will eventually slip out into the right atrium as soon as the balloon is deflated. Eighty percent of patients who had 40-mm device embolization in this series had deficiency of inferior caval and or posterior margins. A snare technique (to hold the screw of the right disc) was sometimes used to hold the device

before deployment as a fall-back option. Inferior vena caval margin is a crucial determinant of device stability, and the margin close to coronary sinus is rarely deficient in published series. In many cases, transesophageal echo can show only absence or presence of a margin; it cannot provide accurate information about the strength of the margin.

Modified techniques as described were used in successful delivery of the device in 82% of cases.[4,5] This was similar to our findings earlier in a retrospective cohort. The deployment technique was modified at the discretion of the operator, to orient the left atrial disc parallel to the septum, with some operators preferring the pulmonary vein technique over the balloon-assisted technique and vice versa.[6] We predominantly used balloon-assistance and pulmonary vein techniques in our patients. This was a not in a randomized manner. However, we found that many patients in the larger atrial septal defect group required more than one technique to receive the overall success of 82% that we recorded. More often than not many anatomic complexities coexisted. Multiple techniques were used on 82 patients out of 346 (23%). In patients in whom balloon assistance failed, 50% had a smaller left atrium, which precluded optimal balloon expansion and opening of the left atrial side of the device. We found that the roof method, dilator assistance and modified sheath offered success in 8/13 of such patients. Irrespective of type of modified techniques, an absent or deficient inferior vena caval or posterior margin and a very large sized defect predicted failure.[4]

The balloon-assisted technique was the most successful technique in our experience (87%). In our opinion, it gives the operator better control of device delivery in all almost morphological variations, such as deficient inferior rim, deficient posterior rim and septal malalignment. The only drawback we find is that it incurs additional vascular access and added expense on the balloon and accessories. Additionally in cases where the left atrium is very small it fails to accommodate the balloon, as described earlier. The left atrial roof method and dilator-assisted support methods were used in only a very few cases with relatively small left atriums, after the balloon technique failed. The pulmonary vein technique was useful for posterior malalignment and septal aneurysm cases. The technique had a success rate of 67%, but in our opinion it requires a steeper learning curve in the release of the left atrial disc that is supposed to stretch across the defect into right atrium after getting anchored to the pulmonary vein origin. In cases where the left atrial dimensions are long, the whole right atrial disc tends to get deployed in the left atrium, causing failure of the technique. Furthermore, the initiation of the left disc delivery deep inside the pulmonary vein ostium may cause failure of the disc to get released out of the ostium.

REFERENCES

1. Amin Z. Trans catheter closure of secundum atrial septal defects. *Catheter Cardiovasc Interv.* 2006; 68(5):778–87.
2. Jung SY, Choi JY. Transcatheter closure of atrial septal defect: Principles and available devices. *J Thorac Dis.* 2018; 10(Suppl 24):S2909–22.
3. Dalvi BV, Pinto RJ, Gupta A. New technique for device closure of large atrial septal defects. *Catheter Cardiovasc Interv.* 2005; 64(1):102–7.
4. Pillai AA, Satheesh S, Pakkirisamy G, Selvaraj R, Jayaraman B. Techniques and outcomes of transcatheter closure of complex atrial septal defects—Single center experience. *Indian Heart J.* 2014; 66(1):38–44.
5. Pillai AA, Sinouvassalou S, Jagadessan KS. Spectrum of morphological abnormalities and treatment outcomes in ostium secundum type of atrial septal defects: Single center experience in >500 cases. *J Saudi Heart Assoc.* 2019; 31(1):12–23.
6. Pillai AA, Rangaswamy Balasubramanian V, Selvaraj R, Saktheeswaran M, Satheesh S, Jayaraman B. Utility of balloon assisted technique in trans catheter closure of very large (≥35 mm) atrial septal defects. *Cardiovasc Diagn Ther.* 2014; 4(1):21–27.

10

Surgical closure techniques

A HANDA, S GOUSY

Surgical correction is the standard of care for ASDs other than secundum defects, such as ostium primum and sinus venosus ASDs. The surgical approach was previously the standard of care for even ostium secundum defects, proving to be both safe and effective. However, over the past few decades many devices have been developed to treat secundum ASD percutaneously, and the benefits of the percutaneous approach have been well demonstrated in both paediatric and young population.[1] Most operators agree that the majority of secundum ASDs can be closed percutaneously. When it is not feasible, the surgical approach is still recommended. Issues such as a defect size of >40 mm and lack of adequate rims of tissue from the defects to important surrounding structures, atrial thrombus and contraindication to antiplatelet therapy are in this category.[2]

The presence of other congenital cardiac deformities such as anomalous pulmonary venous drainage, ostium primum, sinus venosus or coronary sinus ASD are also definite indications for surgical correction of the atria septal defects.

Surgical closure was previously the standard treatment for ASD closure but has now been mostly replaced by the percutaneous approach, albeit in some conditions it still remains the only option as listed above. Also, the standard midline thoracotomy was the preferred approach in ASD surgery, but now most surgeons prefer the minimally invasive right thoracotomy.

SURGICAL CLOSURE

Patients are supported by a heart-lung machine intraoperatively, and the ASD is approached through an opening in the right atrium[3] (Figure 10.1).

Smaller ASDs can be closed by simply using a suture and overseeing the defect. For larger ASDs, a patch is usually used to close the defect. This patch can be taken from the pericardium or made from synthetic materials such as Dacron or Teflon[3] (Figure 10.2).

Most ASDs can be corrected using the minimally invasive surgical approach. Instead of the traditional large midline-incision followed by the division of sternum used in open surgery in the past era, surgeons now perform the procedure by making a small 4- to 5-cm incision on the right side of the chest, reducing the complications and making it a cosmetically feasible procedure (Figure 10.3).

The patient is temporarily put on a heart-lung machine which is usually accessed and inserted via a small incision in the groin, for allowing the sewing of the patch in place. The surgery is performed through the space between the ribs. A retractor is inserted, which gently opens the narrow space between the ribs, enabling the surgeon to insert the specialized, minimally invasive instruments. An endoscope, ideally with a 3D camera, is inserted that provides a high-resolution image of the heart and the ASD (Figure 10.4).

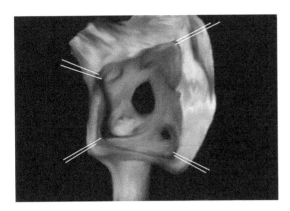

Figure 10.1 ASD approached through an opening in the right atrium. (Illustration by Saranya Gousy.)

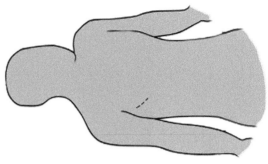

Figure 10.3 Illustration of the now commonly used small 4- to 5-cm incision on the right side of the chest, instead of the large midline incision and division of the sternum used previously in open surgery. (Illustration by Saranya Gousy.)

With this technique, the stability of the chest is fully preserved, the patient recovers faster and the small scar is barely visible after the patient recovers.

Many studies have compared surgical procedure with the transcatheter intervention and have mostly shown equivalent results. A recent randomised controlled trial (RCT) in 2016 of 4606 transcatheter procedures and 3159 surgeries at 35 children's hospitals showed that both transcatheter and surgical ASD closure had excellent short-term outcomes, but transcatheter procedures had shorter lengths of stay and lower rates of infection and complications, resulting in lower overall costs. For children who are eligible, transcatheter ASD closure provides better short-term value than surgery.[4]

Conventional surgery

Ostium Secundum-ASD was conventionally closed through a median sternotomy. Alternative approaches for closure were right anterolateral (peri-aeriolar) thoracotomy and lower mini-sternotomy. The technique chosen was either a direct or patch (autologous pericardium, Dacron, PTFE, bovine pericardium) closure depending upon the size, shape and location of the defect.

After midline sternotomy, the thymus is divided and the pericardial patch is harvested. The patch is either treated with glutaraldehyde. On systemic heparinization and aorto-bicaval cannulation, cardiopulmonary bypass is established and patient is cooled to 32°C. Superior vena caval cannulation is done through the right atrial appendage. In atrial

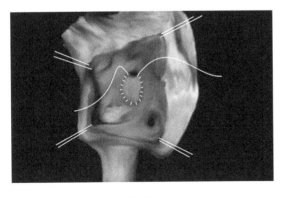

Figure 10.2 Closure of ASD using patch (pericardial patch or Dacron/Teflon patch) (Illustration by Saranya Gousy.)

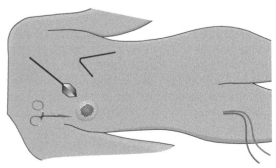

Figure 10.4 Transcatheter ASD closure technique. (Illustration by Saranya Gousy.)

septal defects with deficient inferior rim, selective inferior vena caval cannulation is done as cannulation high in the right atrium, which makes patch closure difficult as cannula will come on the way while taking suture bites inferiorly. Cold-blood cardioplegia is delivered through the aortic root and the heart is arrested. After the caval snares are tightened, the right atrium is opened obliquely, from the right atrial appendage towards the inferior vena cava. Left atrial venting is done directly across the defect, and the anatomy is inspected for normal pulmonary and systemic venous drainage, right ventricular outflow tract obstruction and mitral and tricuspid regurgitation.

In cases of septal aneurysm with fossa ovalis ASD, the aneurysmal septum is excised due to risk of thrombogenicity if plicated. In case of fenestrations associated with a defect, the fenestrated septum is also excised to make it a single defect so that the margins of the defect are strong enough to hold the suture. The coronary sinus, septal tricuspid annulus and the tendon of Todaro form the triangle of Koch, which is the location of AV node. This is identified, and the suture bites are taken closer on the antero-inferior rim so as to avoid the AV node. In a deficient inferior rim and selective IVC cannulation, suture bites are taken onto the floor of the left atrium. The eustachian valve should not be mistaken for the inferior rim, as suturing the patch to the eustachian valve will result in directing the IVC blood to left atrium.

The patch is seated to the inferior rim first, using running proline sutures, and then the suturing is carried on to the anterior and posterior rim and then finally to the superior rim. Valsalva manoeuvre is performed before tying the knot to fill the left atrium with blood, which will prevent any air embolism. Additional valve repair procedures are carried out if planned. The right atrium is closed and then the snuggers are loosened. The aortic cross clamp is released and the heart weaned off cardiopulmonary bypass.[3]

Surgery versus device closure

While surgery continues to be gold standard in the treatment of OS-ASD as it can deal with all the morphological variations, catheter closure requires detailed imaging protocol before attempting. Device stability is highly dependent on morphological features such as size of the defect, size of the selected device, adequacy of rims and proximity to structures such as the AV node, inferior vena cava and mitral annulus. Catheter intervention in complex defects is plagued by issues such as device embolization and device erosion. A surgical approach is definitely more invasive, but is free of the device-related issues mentioned before. Both forms of therapy have established their role in the clinical practice. Both techniques have evolved with time as well. Modified trans catheter closure (TCC) techniques offer improved closure rates in a catheterization laboratory, thus reducing surgical referrals. Surgical incisions have become minimal, reducing post-operative morbidity.[4]

Our data, involving more than 500 cases in single-centre registry, shows that outcomes of TCC and invasive surgical ASD repair are similar overall, with no significant differences seen in functional outcomes or number of residual shunts. Although residual shunts in particular trended higher with TCC, these tended to be mild, clinically insignificant shunts that did not result in a difference in functional status. We found similar outcomes with different surgical approaches (conventional sternotomy and minimally invasive incisions). The number of peri-procedural complications was low in both groups, and it is expected to be difficult to show a significant difference between the groups. Length of stay in hospital and ICU was much shorter for TCC. However, this immediate benefit was balanced by a trend towards higher residual shunts in TCC. Late device migration or embolization is always a concern in transcatheter patients, although we did not see any such events in early follow-up. Delayed device erosion and embolization remains a possibility. Both surgical and transcatheter techniques have evolved over time. Studies conducted in previous decades have shown excellent long-term outcomes with the conventional midline sternotomy approach. Later on, modified approaches such as anterolateral and mini sternotomies were shown to be equally efficient to less-invasive strategies. About 45% of our surgical patients underwent one of the modified approaches. The surgical outcomes were not influenced by the defect anatomy, while TCC had anatomical predictors for failure. The heart team approach is important in planning the best treatment strategy in a given anatomy.

REFERENCES

1. Butera G, Carminati M, Chessa M, et al. Percutaneous versus surgical closure of secundum atrial septal defect: Comparison of early results and complications. *Am Heart J.* 2006; 151(1):228–234.

2. Siddiqui WT, Usman T, Atiq M, Amanullah MM. Transcatheter versus surgical closure of atrial septum defect: A debate from A developing country. *J Cardiovasc Thorac Res.* 2014; 6(4):205–210.

3. Hopkins RA, Bert AA, Buchholz B, Guarino K, Meyers M. Surgical patch closure of atrial septal defects. *Ann Thorac Surg.* 2004; 77(6):2144–2150.

4. Du ZD, Hijazi ZM, Kleinman CS, Silverman NH, Larntz K. Amplatzer investigators. Comparison between transcatheter and surgical closure of secundum atrial septal defect in children and adults: Results of a multicenter nonrandomized trial. *J Am Coll Cardiol.* 2002; 39(11):1836–1844.

11

Transcatheter closure of complex and large ASDs

A A PILLAI, V BALASUBRAMANIAN

Transcatheter closure of atrial septal defects (ASDs) has become standard therapy in the management of most of ostium secundum ASDs. It can be safely performed with excellent results when appropriate techniques are used. Most ASDs (25–75%) are centrally located and closure of the defects is straightforward. But a considerable percentage has complex anatomy which is challenging to close percutaneously. ASDs that are difficult to close percutaneously may be large, have deficient rims, be aneurysmal or have multiple fenestrated defects. These defects are termed 'complex' ASDs.[1]

In a study by Pedra et al., complex ASDs were defined as ASD with complex anatomy such as the presence of large ASDs (stretched diameter more than 26 mm); ASDs associated with deficient rims (≤4 mm) at anterior, inferior or posterior portion; two separate ASDs within the septum; multifenestrated ASDs; ASDs with floppy redundant and hypermobile septum (excursion ≥10 mm) considered to be aneurysmal or combination of these. The success of complex ASD closure mainly relies on proper pre-procedural imaging techniques.[2] Morphology of atrial septum is paramount in any closure of complex ASDs. Complex anatomy, especially sinusoidal defects and fenestrated defects, needs careful assessment prior to the procedure.

LARGE DEFECTS

Large ASDs even with adequate rims are complex ASDs. ASDs with stretched diameter larger than 26 mm are considered to be large. Although closure would appear to be a simple procedure, the size of device to be used to close such defects remains to be determined. There are other issues, such as whether the left atrium would accommodate large discs fear of impingement of the device on adjacent structures such as the aorta pulmonary veins causing obstruction, mitral valve and vena cava. Large defects are associated with deficient rims, which make device closure still challenging.

Deficient septal rims

An adequate rim is 7 mm or larger. A deficient rim is less than 3 mm. Inadequate rims are between 3 and 5 mm. To close the ASDs the operator should have thorough knowledge of atrial septal rims and adjoining structures. With minor modification to the classification proposed by Shrivastava and Radhakrishnan, Amin et al. has as in Figure 11.1 suggested[3]

1. Aortic rim—rim adjacent to aortic valve
2. SVC (superior vena cava) rim—rim adjacent to SVC
3. Superior rim—rim between aortic rim and SVC rim
4. Posterior rim—rim opposite to aortic rim
5. IVC (inferior vena cava) rim—rim adjacent to IVC
6. Atrioventricular rim—rim adjacent to AV valve.

Deficient antero-superior rims

Deficient antero-superior rims are associated with large ASDs. In our centre largest ASDs had deficient antero-superior rims. The main problem with a deficient antero-superior rim is that during the transcatheter closure there is the problem of straddling the left atrial disc on the aorta, which can lead to erosion of the device. Initial reports of device erosion have led to use of oversizing the device by 4 mm more than the stretched diameter so that the device remains flared to prevent any discrete area of pressure on aorta where erosion may occur. The other frequent problem is that

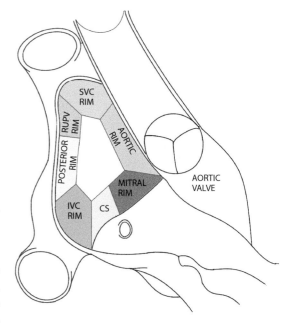

Figure 11.1 Classification of atrial septal rims. Illustration depicts different rims of ostium secundum ASDs. CS: coronary sinus, RUPV: right upper pulmonary vein, SVC: superior vena cava, IVC: inferior vena cava. (Illustration by Saranya Gousy.)

larger the LA disc, the more perpendicular it lies to the septal defect and may prolapse into the RA. So modified techniques have been developed, such as the Hausdorf sheath technique which uses a specially designed sheath with two curves which helps in aligning the disc parallel to the septum during deployment.

Deficient posterior or postero-inferior rims

Closure of large ASDs with posterior rim is real challenge. As the difference in the radial length between right and left disc is 3 mm, deficient rims will not allow the ASD device to be stable. This leads to complications such as device embolization and impingement of the device on adjacent structures.

Multiple or fenestrated discs

Multiple ASDs account for 13% of all of secundum ASDs. They are complex defects that may be successfully closed by more than one device.

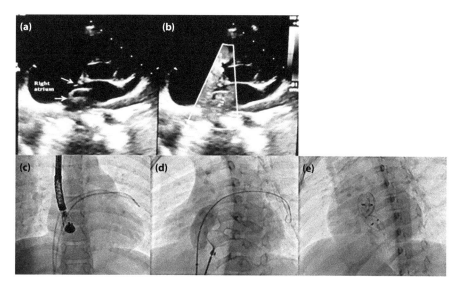

Figure 11.2 TEE images showing device closure in fenestrated ASDs (a, b) and balloon assistance for closing multiple ASDs (c–e).

If the distance between two defects is less than 7 mm, closing the larger defect will close the smaller defects too. If the distance is more than 7 mm, then echocardiographic evaluation with balloon occlusion of larger defects will help in deciding whether to use two devices.[7] If the smaller defect is significant it should be closed prior to closing the larger defect as shown in Figure 11.2.

Atrial septal aneurysm

Large defects have septal excursions of more than 10 mm, which are termed septal aneurysms and make device closure quite challenging. Double disc devices such as the Helex buttoned device or the Amplatzer cribriform device are appropriate choices. Zomara et al. successfully closed defects associated with large septal aneurysms with buttoned devices by compressing the aneurismal tissue between occluder and counteroccluder.

BALLOON SIZING THE DEFECT

Balloon sizing of large ASDs is a useful method as most ASDs are not circular. They are oval in shape, and selecting the correct size is challenging. Some of the sizing balloons available are from companies like NUmed, Amplatzer and Cocoon.[2] Usually they are available in 18-, 24-, 34-mm sizes only. These balloons are compliant and soft so they

can stretch and increase the size of the defect and falsify the actual defect size. Some operators do not use this method for fear of complications. Amin et al. have recommended the stop-flow technique when balloon sizing is done. In this method, the sizing balloon is kept across the ASD and inflated with saline contrast mixture; colour Doppler echo confirms the disappearance of the shunt. This is followed by deflation until the shunt reappears and then inflation just till the shunt disappears. This is the stop-flow diameter of the ASD. A device equal to or 2 mm larger than the stop-flow diameter is usually chosen. This is difficult in cases of malaligned septum and in small children with larger defects as it can obstruct the inflow portion and lead to hypotension.

TECHNIQUES EMPLOYED FOR COMPLEX ASD DEVICE CLOSURE

Transcatheter closure of complex ASDs is usually challenging. Some modified techniques are available based on the operator's choice and experience in using those methods. In the case of complex ASDs, the spectrum of anatomic variation is high, and this may challenge the success of the procedure and sometimes complicate the transcatheter closure and pose a risk of device embolization. Understanding the morphological anatomy is the basis of the transcatheter closure success.[3] The size of the defect, location and boundaries or margins of the defect have to be clearly understood by imaging before attempting the closure. A large ostium secundum ASD of more than 20 mm in a child and more than 30 mm in an adult is always a concern because these are the defects which have deficient margins; these always require some modification from routine technique, and defects more than 40 mm require a custom-made device and have a higher risk of failure.

Rims are defined with standard descriptions. A deficient rim is one which is less than 5 mm. The rims measured also do not tell the real strength with which the device is being held. The following rims, shown in Figure 11.3, must be looked at in detail before the procedure:

1. The antero-superior rim or the Aortic rim
2. The antero-inferior rim or the AV valve rim
3. The postero-superior rim or the SVC rim
4. The postero-inferior rim or the IVC rim
5. The true posterior/RUPV rim.

Several morphological complexities that can pose challenges during the procedure are large ASDs (≥30 mm), multiple ASDs, aneurysmal septum, malalignment of septum, rim deficiency or floppiness. Podnar et al. in his article has described common morphological variations in OS-ASD: deficient rim (Figure 11.4) is retroaortic rim (42.1%), deficient infero-posterior rim (12.1%), perforated aneurysm of the septum (7.9%), multiple defects (7.3%), combined deficiency of mitral and aortic rims (4.1%), deficient SVC rim (1%) and deficient coronary sinus rim (1%).[3]

In our centre the morphological variations studied by TEE (Figure 11.5), which were major causes of transcatheter closure failure, were deficient IVC/posterior rim and defects more than 35 mm in size. The success rate of transcatheter closure in complex ASDs in our centre was 91%. Our experience has shown that the deficient aortic rim does not represent absolute contraindication for transcatheter closure.[4] Even though by convention deficient rims are considered to be less than 5 mm and the value is arbitrary, the strength of

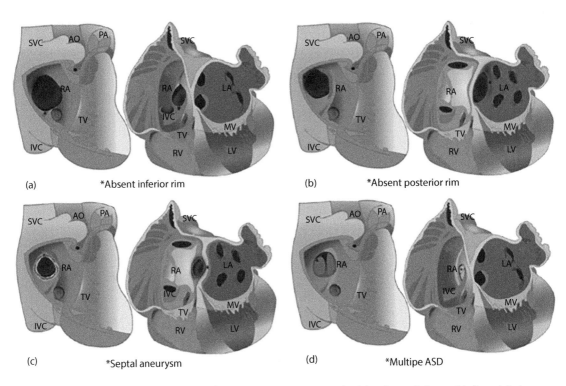

(a) *Absent inferior rim

(b) *Absent posterior rim

(c) *Septal aneurysm

(d) *Multipe ASD

Figure 11.3 Pictorial representation of various anatomic complexities from right and left atrial views. Absent IVC rim **(a)**, absent posterior rim **(b)**, septal aneurysm **(c)**, multiple ASD **(d)**. SVC: superior vena cava, IVC: inferior vena cava, RA: right atrium, LA: left atrium, TV: tricuspid valve, LV: left ventricle, RV: right ventricle.

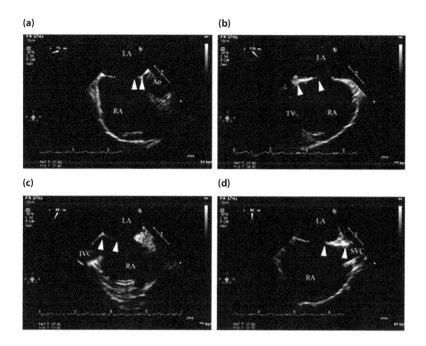

Figure 11.4 Distance between arrowheads is measured as length of a rim. TEE images at 15 showing a deficient aortic rim (a), at 135 showing an AVV rim (b), at 60 showing an IVC rim (c) and at 90 showing an SVC rim.

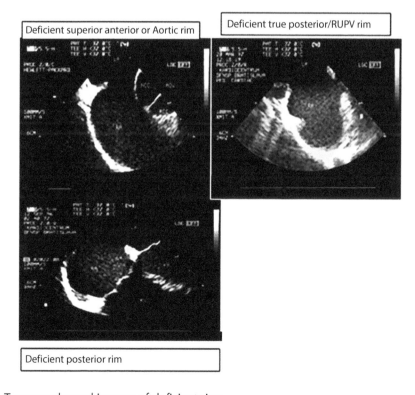

Figure 11.5 Transesophageal images of deficient rims.

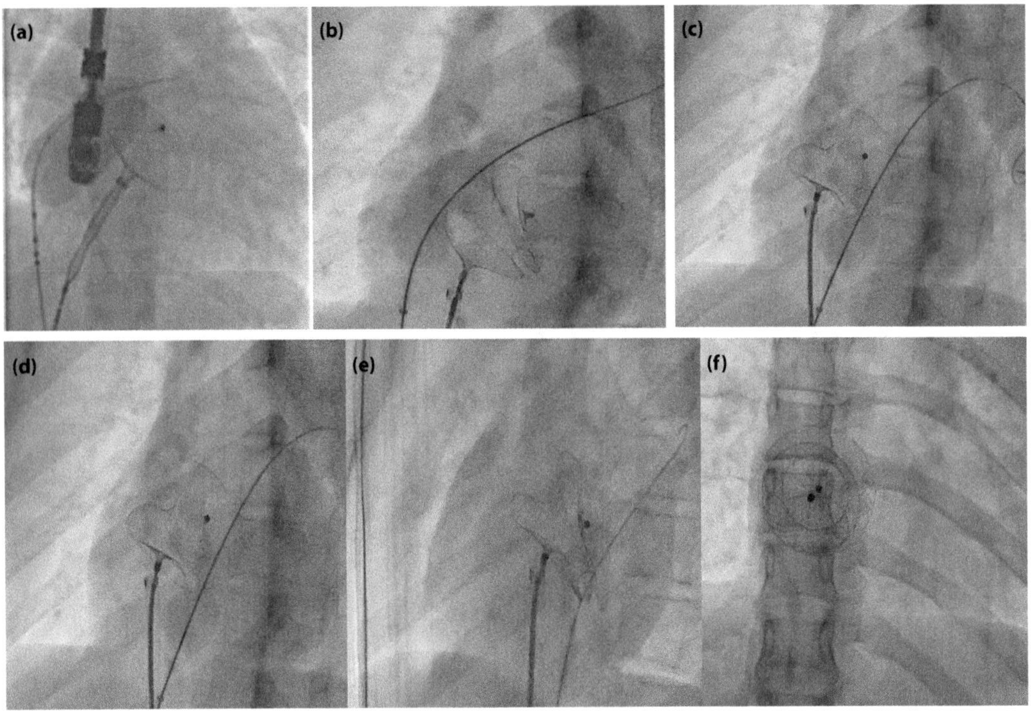

Figure 11.6 Serial fluoroscopic images of balloon-assisted device closure of a large 38.5-mm atrial septal defect with a 42-mm ASD device (a–f). Left disc being delivered with balloon inflated across the defect (a); whole device delivered with balloon inflated, device assuming an hour-glass shape with waist being compressed by the balloon (b); the waist expands as balloon starts deflating (c); the waist expands further as balloon gets smaller (d); device in good position after complete deflation (e); deployed after withdrawal of the balloon (f).

rim is more important than the length. Also the location of the defect is important, with ellipsoid peripheral location posing more challenges than the central oval defect. By modified techniques our success rate was 79%.

Some of the modified techniques[4] are as follows:

1. Balloon-assisted technique
2. Pulmonary vein deployment method
3. Combination of two different techniques
4. LA roof method
5. Modified sheath method
6. Multiple devices with balloon-occlusion technique

Balloon-assisted technique

With the help of a contralateral venous sheath a compliant sizing balloon—either Amplatzer or Cocoon balloon measuring 24 mm and 34 mm—was used to occlude the defect partially or fully, supporting

the device delivery.[2,6] The device is delivered from left or right upper pulmonary vein with the balloon over the wire placed on contralateral side. With the balloon in the inflated position, the LA disc is deployed, the sheath is withdrawn and the RA disc is released. Then the balloon is deflated slowly and the balloon and the wire are removed meticulously with TEE guidance (Figure 11.7), ensuring alignment of the device discs on either side of the septum as shown in Figure 11.6.

Pulmonary vein deployment technique

In this method, as shown in Figures 11.8 and 11.9, the LA disc is partially deployed in either the left or right upper pulmonary vein, creating an American football–like appearance. Momentary release of LA disc is done when the RA disc stretches out to catch the two sides of septum. Here the sheath is kept stable until the RA disc is deployed, simultaneously

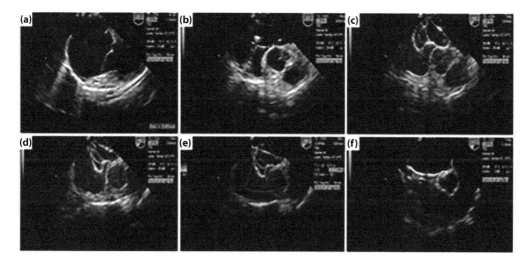

Figure 11.7 Serial transesophageal images of balloon-assisted technique for 38.5-mm defect closed by 42-mm device, showing large ASD of 38.5 mm with deficient posterior rim (a), sizing balloon occluding the defect (b), hourglass-shaped device with waist compressed by balloon (c), balloon deflated and waist expanded (d), device snuggly fitting (e), and after removal of balloon (f).

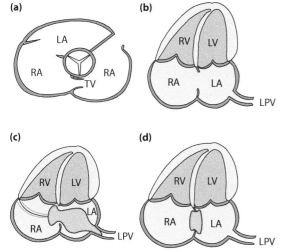

Figure 11.8 Pulmonary vein deployment technique.

pulling down the LA disc as both discs catch the septum simultaneously. This technique is usually used in cases with deficient antero-superior rims. Care should be taken not to deep seat the device into the pulmonary vein or cause injury.

Left atrial roof deployment technique

In patients with deficient aortic and posterior rims and a small atrial cavity, the left atrial disc is large enough so that it protrudes into the right atrium and precludes successful procedure. In this situation, a left atrial roof method can be used. Here the LA disc is opened against the LA roof before deployment, as shown in Figure 11.10. The delivery sheath is placed in the orifice of the upper pulmonary vein and not into the vein. The sheath is stabilized against the LA roof and then slowly withdrawn when the RA disc is deployed. This

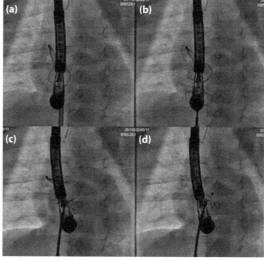

Figure 11.9 Fluoroscopic images of right upper pulmonary vein technique.

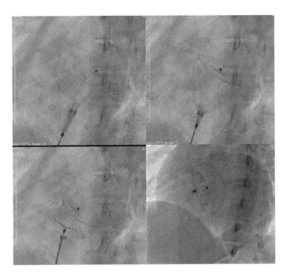

Figure 11.10 LA disc is placed near the orifice of pulmonary vein near the roof of the left atrium and not inside pulmonary vein, and right atrial disc is deployed as shown (a–d).

manoeuvre keeps the LA disc inside the atrial cavity and prevents a prolapse into the right atrium.

Modified cut-sheath approach

The operator cuts the sheath tip in an oblique fashion to allow for asymmetric expansion of the left atrial disc to catch the rims with simultaneous deployment of right sided disc. This technique is used in defects with a malaligned septum.

Bousfield-Spies technique

In this method, a bevel is placed at inner curvature of a 12-F Cook sheath so that the outlet orientation is sideways, making a parallel orientation to the septum. This technique was used to close large ASDs by Dr Christian Bousfield and Dr Spies.

SSH technique or Kutty method

This technique was used in closing large ASDs with deficient inferior and antero-superior rims. Here the Mullins transseptal sheath is modified. A Mullins transseptal sheath 2-F, larger than the ASD device, is cut at delivery end so that tip is straight but opening is sideways. Once the device is released, it gets oriented parallel to the septum for device closure.

Nounou Agilis method

This is a novel technique in which a steerable electrophysiology catheter Agilis catheter (St. Jude Medical Inc., Minneapolis, Minnesota) is used. The curved sheath is advanced into LA such that the device is oriented parallel to septum and deployed. In this method, devices larger than 20 mm cannot be used.

Wahab technique/dilator-assisted technique

In this technique, two femoral venous sheaths are used where a 0.035″ wire is advanced to the end of dilator, which is advanced into the left atrium and manoeuvred to hold the left atrial disc parallel to the septum as shown in (Figure 11.11). The dilator and wire are removed once the device is deployed. This is used in patients with large ASDs with deficient anterior or posterior rims.

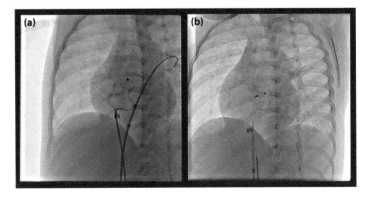

Figure 11.11 Dilator with wire inside for stabilizing the LA disc in Wahab technique.

Parallel wire technique

Here a soft 0.018" wire is used just to maintain access to the LA in case of multiple small ASDs and not for stabilizing the device.

Goose neck snare technique

In this method, a 5-mm goose neck snare with 4-Fr catheter is advanced up to the screwing mechanism of the device in parallel.[5] When the delivery cable is unscrewed and the final device position is satisfactory, the goose sneck snare is released by opening the loop. If the position is not satisfactory the device is snared and repositioned again.

Hausdorf sheath technique

This technique was used in cases where large ASDs have deficient anterior or antero-superior rims. It is a special sheath with two posterior curves and an angled tip which helps in keeping the device parallel to the septum during deployment and away from the aortic mound. This sheath is available from Cook Medical in 10-F, 11-F and 12-F sizes.

The main objective of various deployment techniques is to orient the left atrial disc parallel to the septum with any single technique, such as the balloon-assisted technique, pulmonary vein technique or a combination of both as shown in Figure 11.12.[4] The left atrial roof technique was selected were the balloon-assisted or pulmonary vein technique failed. The cut-sheath method was used when the retroaortic margin was deficient

and where conventional methods failed. Size alone was not the criterion for deciding surgical method, but large defects have associated complexities, such as malaligned septum or deficient rims, which may reduce the success of transcatheter closure. The posterior or inferior IVC rims are important for holding the device, and their deficiency makes the patient a candidate for surgical closure. Combined rim deficiency is seen where both the IVC rim and anterior rim are deficient, making transcatheter closure difficult. On rare occasions coronary sinus rim deficiency is seen, which makes surgery the only option.

COMPLICATIONS OF TRANSCATHETER DEVICE CLOSURE

Complications arising due to transcatheter closure are rare but lethal in a minority of cases. Device embolization, device erosion, cardiac tamponade and cardiac death are some of the major complications arising from transcatheter device closure of ASD. Compared to surgical closure, transcatheter closure is associated with lower morbidity and fewer complications. Globally minor complications occur in 5% of cases and major complications in 1–3%. The US FDA and the Manufacturer and User Facility Device Experience (MAUDE) database has shown similar mortality between surgical and transcatheter device closure. But emergency surgical approaches have shown 20-fold higher mortality in device-related adverse effects. Major complications occurred more in the surgical group than with transcatheter closure. Device embolization occurs in approximately 0.1–0.4% of cases, particularly with ASD closure devices. Device embolization is a potential life-threatening complication, requiring immediate removal by either percutaneous or surgical intervention.

Risk factors

Meta-analysis studies have shown several risk factors linked to device-related adverse effects. Patients may present with haemodynamic instability to ventricular fibrillation due to various causes such as cardiac tamponade, free wall rupture, LVOT obstruction and coronary artery compression. Older age, morphology and size of the defect, size of the device (either under or oversized) and the expertise of the centre are related to adverse effects.

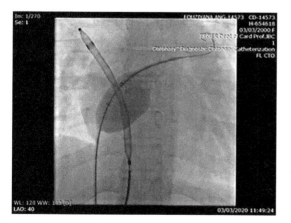

Figure 11.12 Combined balloon-assisted and pulmonary vein deployment technique.

Device embolization

Large and complex ASDs pose problems during transcatheter device closure. In case of large ASDs, deficient rims may pose special problems, leading to device undersizing and device embolization. Device malposition and embolization occur in large ASDs, especially more than 35 mm. Deficient inferior/posterior rims have higher risk for embolization. Deficient antero-superior rims are not a problem for embolization, but an oversized device may lead to device embolization as in Figure 11.13. In the case of large ASDs with aneurysms, device closure becomes even more challenging.

Management of device embolization

Successful transcatheter closure requires meticulous planning and adequate knowledge of the risk factors, such as large defects, deficient rims, undersizing the defect leading to mismatched device because of faulty interpretation of the imaging, which may lead to catastrophic consequences. Usually a device embolizes in the pulmonary artery (Figure 11.13) and very rarely has been retrieved from the aorta or iliac arteries. Availability of retrieval tools and multimodality imaging such as 3D echo and bi-plane fluoroscopy,

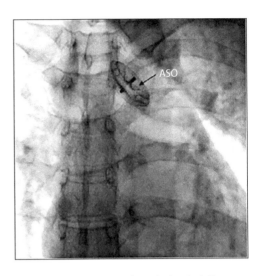

Figure 11.13 Atrial septal occluder (ASO) embolized to pulmonary artery.

not only facilitates snaring the embolized device but provides a real-time survey of damage to surrounding structures.

Self-made snares like 0.014″ coronary wires, 0.032″ Teflon wires through 5-F or 6-F guide catheters can be used to snare the devices (Figure 11.14). Percutaneous snare techniques are always attempted first if the patient is haemodynamically stable and care is taken to avoid damage to adjacent valvular, vascular and conduction

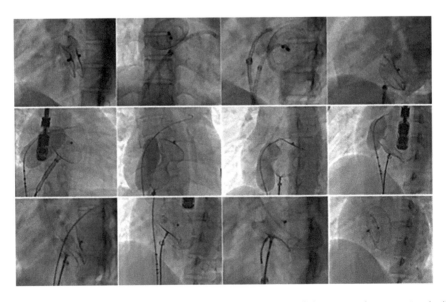

Figure 11.14 Snaring of embolized ASD device and deployment of the same device using balloon-assisted technique.

system structures.[3,4] Goose neck snares, multi-loop snares and Ensnares are used for retrieving an embolized device by catching the central pin or the device itself by using a larger snare.[4] Non-snare devices such as bioptomes, forcep devices, electrical mapping catheter systems or interventional radiology systems like basket retrieval systems can be used. If percutaneous technique has failed, or if there is haemodynamic instability, then a surgical option can be tried.

Device erosion

Device erosion, although rare, can occur after device implantation either immediately during first 3 days or several months later. Erosion can occur through the atrial free wall or through the aortic wall, causing pericardial effusion, haemopericardium with tamponade and death if not treated. Diagnosis is usually made by serial echo or cardiac CT, which can differentiate between inflammatory reaction or true erosion. Device sizing by multimodality imaging helps in correct sizing of the device and can prevent this dreaded complication.

Arrhythmias

Atrial arrhythmias, SVT, AV blocks and rarely ventricular tachycardia and ventricular fibrillation have been reported. Atrial fibrillation has been reported to increase after device closure, especially in elderly patients and patients with large defects, but large studies are lacking to support this notion. Contradictory accounts report decreases in the overall incidence of atrial fibrillation. Transient AV blocks, ranging from first degree to complete AV blocks, have been reported to occur in 1–6% reported immediately to 2–3 weeks later, but the requirement of a permanent pacemaker is very rare.

Other complications

Reports of rare occurrence of aortic incompetence caused by traction on noncoronary cusps due to tissue endothelialization and fibrosis have been seen, but the severity of aortic regurgitation is usually mild to moderate and does not warrant any intervention. Coronary compression can occur due to an abnormal course of the left circumflex artery arising from the right coronary sinus due to a large disc causing external compression. New onset migraine has been reported in 8–10% of the patients post ASD device closure, but the real underlying mechanism is not established and they have good response to dual antiplatelet therapy. Thrombosis of the left side disc has been reported, but long-term anticoagulation has not been required in most cases.

CONCLUSION

During the past decade the transcatheter technique has become the default method for ASD closure. The crux of success lies in meticulous pre-procedural imaging and understanding the anatomy, especially in complex ASDs as successful transcatheter procedure provides equal efficacy, fewer complications, lower cost and shorter hospital stays compared to surgical closure methods.

REFERENCES

1. Suárez De Lezo J, Medina A, Pan M, et al. Transcatheter occlusion of complex atrial septal defects. *Catheter Cardiovasc Interv.* 2000; 51(1):33–41.
2. Sobrino A, Basmadjian AJ, Ducharme A, et al. Multiplanar transesophageal echocardiography for the evaluation and percutaneous management of ostium secundum atrial septal defects in the adult. *Arch Cardiol Mex.* 2012; 82(1):37–47.
3. Pillai AA, Rangaswamy Balasubramanian V, Selvaraj R, Saktheeswaran M, Satheesh S, Jayaraman B. Utility of balloon assisted technique in trans catheter closure of very large (≥35 mm) atrial septal defects. *Cardiovasc Diagn Ther.* 2014; 4(1):21–27.
4. Pillai AA, Sinouvassalou S, Jagadessan KS, Munuswamy H. Spectrum of morphological abnormalities and treatment outcomes in ostium secundum type of atrial septal defects: Single center experience in >500 cases. *J Saudi Heart Assoc.* 2019; 31(1):12–23.
5. Pillai AA, Satheesh S, Pakkirisamy G, Selvaraj R, Jayaraman B. Techniques and outcomes of transcatheter closure

of complex atrial septal defects—single center experience. *Indian Heart J*. 2014; 66(1):38–44.

6. Pillai AA, Upadhyay A, Gousy S, Handa A. Impact of modified techniques of transcatheter closure in large atrial septal defects (≥30 mm) with anatomic complexities. *Cardiol Young*. 2018; 28(10):1122–33.

7. Butera G, Lovin N, Paola Basile D, Carminati M. Goose-neck snare-assisted transcatheter ASD closure: A safety procedure for large and complex ASDs. *Catheter Cardiovasc Interv*. 2016; 87(5):926–30.

8. Dalvi BV, Pinto RJ, Gupta A. New technique for device closure of large atrial septal defects. *Catheter Cardiovasc Interv*. 2005; 64(1):102–7.

9. Lander SR, Phillips S, Vallabhan RC, Grayburn PA, Anwar A. Percutaneous closure of multiple atrial septal defects with three Amplatzer septal occluder devices. *Catheter Cardiovasc Interv*. 2004; 62(4):526–9.

12

Transcatheter closure in special situations

V BALASUBRAMANIAN

ASDs often are not detected until late adulthood. Many patients present as elderly adults with significantly large ASDs. The incidence of congenital heart disease is increasingly detected in the adult population; also, children with congenital heart disease are living into adulthood. Large ASDs are associated with significant morbidity and mortality as mortality increases with increasing age. Campbell et al. reported increasing mortality with increasing age with 0.7% at the second and third decades to 7.6% at the sixth and seventh decades. The increase in mortality is due to pulmonary hypertension and right-heart failure. Murphy et al. reported that patients operated before 25 years of age had similar life expectancy to matched controls, whereas those operated later in life had poor outcomes.[1,2]

TRANSCATHETER CLOSURE IN ELDERLY

In elderly patients with large ASDs, the most common symptom is effort-induced dyspnoea. This is usually not disabling, and the majority continue with normal activity. Clinical disability increases with age, and major difficulty arises after 60 years.[4] Even though there is not a direct correlation between shunt size or symptoms and age, development of pulmonary vascular resistance alters the course of ASDs. The disabling symptoms develop due to progressive heart failure, and onset of chronic atrial arrhythmias such as atrial flutter or atrial fibrillation is reported in as many as 52% of patients with uncorrected ASDs. Compared to younger patients, older patients with ASD have a reduced life span. The average age of death is before 50 in patients with untreated large ASDs. The patients die of right-heart failure or pulmonary arterial hypertension. In large ASDs with almost equal atrial pressures, the difference in compliance between the right and left ventricles allows left-to-right shunt. As age increases the left ventricle becomes less compliant and systemic arteriolar elasticity decreases, leading to a rise in systemic vascular resistance, which in turn leads to an increase in left-to-right shunt. Closing this ASD may cut off the pop-off mechanism for the left-to right shunt, leading to an increase in pulmonary congestion and acute pulmonary oedema due to diastolic LV stiffness in the elderly.[3]

Thus in elderly patients, especially those over 60 years, it is generally recommended to occlude the defect with a balloon test for 15–20 minutes and measure the LA pressure. If LA pressure exceeds more than 30–35 mm Hg it can lead to pulmonary venous congestion or pulmonary oedema, suggesting that LV may be too compromised to allow closure of ASD.[4] This is likely to unmask the LV diastolic stiffness, which leads to an increase in LA pressure and further events. Holzer et al. reported a suitable method of closure in these elderly patients by adequately treating systemic hypertension as well providing pre-treatment with diuretics and afterload reducing agents in cases where transient-balloon occlusion caused a temporary increase in LA pressure above the physiologic range; the treatment also includes the use of self-fabricated fenestrated ASD devices for successful closure without causing adverse outcomes with long-term benefits including improvement in diastolic parameters.[4]

In elderly patients with large ASDs, there is an increase in mortality and morbidity.[3,4] Despite controversial reports on mortality after surgical ASD closure, recent reports have shown benefits of either surgical or transcatheter closure of ASD in older patients. Several studies have shown functional improvement after either surgical or percutaneous device closure. Elderly patients with ASD have concomitant cardiac as well as extracardiac pathology, which may affect the surgical outcomes, as well as complications during the perioperative period, involving anaesthesia, sternotomy as well as cardiopulmonary-bypass-related issues. The presence of pulmonary hypertension, large left-to-right shunt, congestive heart failure and/or atrial fibrillation did not affect the surgical short-term or long-term outcomes regardless of age.[5,6] Hence closure of ASD in the elderly is warranted. In comparison to surgical ASD closure, the transcatheter closure is less invasive and patients' functional recovery is faster. The lower morbidity and mortality makes device closure superior where indications of ASD closure are there.

ASD CLOSURE WITH PULMONARY HYPERTENSION

Pulmonary hypertension is a rare but serious complication of ASD. Closure of ASD in such patients warrants caution. Pulmonary arterial hypertension (PAH), defined as mean PA pressure more than 25 mm `, has been noted in 6–35% of patients with ostium secundum ASDs. In large ASDs significant left-to-right shunting is associated with RV volume overload, leading to atrial arrhythmias, pulmonary arterial hypertension and decreased survival. Moderate to severe PAH in large ASDs has been reported in 9–22% of cases.[7] Pulmonary hypertension in unoperated ASD in turn has been associated with right-heart failure, atrial tachyarrhythmia and increase in mortality. PAH in the setting of unoperated ASD can be due to various etiologies. Postcapillary PAH is due to diastolic dysfunction and is usually seen in elderly patients with hypertension, ischaemic heart disease, diabetes mellitus, chronic kidney disease or mitral valve disease. Precapillary PAH is due to either a large shunt or other genetic or associated lung conditions, causing the disproportionate increase in PA pressure to the shunt, or due to irreversible PAH, leading to Eisenmenger syndrome. The hyperkinetic form of PAH in large ASDs, if persistent, will cause muscularization of pulmonary arterioles and can lead to the veno-occlusive type of PAH, which is irreversible.

At one end of the spectrum, there is a group of patients with reversible PAH who will benefit from closure, and at the other end is another group of patients where there is Eisenmengerization, where the closure will be catastrophic. Hence there are patients with large shunt but mild PAH, patients with Eisenmenger syndrome and patients with bystander ASD with severe PAH. Differentiating these conditions requires a multidimensional approach using clinical, electrocardiography, echocardiography, chest X-ray and cardiac catheterization as there are no set guidelines or a specific value of PA pressure to defer ASD closure. During cardiac catheterization, acute vasodilator testing is done and if the pulmonary vascular resistance (PVR) index is less than 6 Woods units or PVR/systemic vascular resistance (SVR) ratio is less than 0.33 then defect closure is considered. Yong et al. study have shown that device closure causes a reduction in PAH severity, but PA pressure may not reach the normal value.[8] There is also an improvement in functional class and a reduction in the incidence of atrial arrhythmias. Balint et al. in their studies have demonstrated a reduction in the incidence of atrial flutter and fibrillation by 41%. Also, they have demonstrated a reduction in PA pressure in both short- and long-term follow-up. Haemodynamic studies measuring PA pressure and left ventricular end-diastolic pressure (LVEDP) in patients with hyperkinetic pulmonary circulation due to large OS-ASD in addition to vasodilator testing will show both short-term and long-term effects on pulmonary vasculature after ASD closure. A >25% decrease in PA pressure during the temporary balloon-occlusion test is considered valid even though the value is arbitrary, and long-term studies are necessary for validity.[8,9]

BALLOON-OCCLUSION TEST

The temporary balloon-occlusion test is done to assess the effect of ASD closure on left ventricular end-diastolic pressure and left atrial pressure in elderly patients with large OS-ASDs and predominant left-to-right shunt with risk factors for diastolic dysfunction such as hypertension and coronary artery disease. It is done to assess the risk of LV heart failure, predominantly diastolic heart function post-ASD closure, even though data supporting the procedure are still lacking. The procedure is done as shown in Figure 12.1 with either the Amplatzer (Abbott, Plymouth, MN) or NuMED (NuMED Inc., Hopkintown, NY) sizing balloon.[10]

During the procedure, left atrial pressure, LVEDP and pulmonary capillary wedge pressure (PCWP) are measured pre- and post-balloon occlusion and an average reading for 6–8 beats is taken. If either baseline LVEDP > 15 mm Hg or post-LA pressure more than 10 mm Hg, LVEDP more than 15 mm Hg then ASD closure is deferred.[9] In patients with suspected diastolic dysfunction and in elderly patients who have poor LV diastolic compliance, ASD may serve as pop-off window and active management of risk factors such as hypertension and coronary artery disease responsible for diastolic dysfunction is required. Also in patients with baseline elevated LA pressure a temporary balloon occlusion will elevate LA pressure and LVEDP if diastolic compliance is poor, especially in patients with hypertension, and will lead to pulmonary oedema and poor outcomes.

FENESTRATED ASD DEVICE CLOSURE

In select patients with pulmonary arterial hypertension with a predominant left-to-right shunting, ASD patients with Down syndrome who may develop pulmonary veno-occlusive disease (PVOD) later in life, or patients with restrictive LV filling, or patients with fenestration, ASD, closure is safe and feasible with either a custom-made or fenestrated ASD device. The use of a fenestrated ASD device closure may be warranted if temporary balloon occlusion for 10–15 minutes shows a rise in LA pressure in case of patients with restrictive LV filling more than physiological range or a rise in PA pressure by more than 5 mm Hg in patients with PAH. Fenestrations are made manually by needle or by passing an 8-F dilator and creating three to five fenestrations, based on the operator, and may act as a pop-off mechanism during a restrictive filling phase both during PAH with right-to-left shunt preventing right-heart volume overload and during diastolic dysfunction with left-to-right shunt preventing pulmonary venous congestion.

PREGNANCY

Pregnancy in a patient with ASD remains uneventful and generally well tolerated. In pregnant patients with ASD, the volume overload on right ventricle is worse, and there is increased incidence of supraventricular tachycardia along with increased risk of thromboembolism. Also patients with incidentally detected ASD tolerate pregnancy well.[11] But pregnant patients with symptoms of pre-existing heart failure do worse and may warrant closure of ASD. Foetal and maternal outcomes are generally good except in patients with severe PAH, where both maternal and foetal outcomes are poor. In addition to the risk of embolism due to atrial arrhythmias in unrepaired ASDs, there

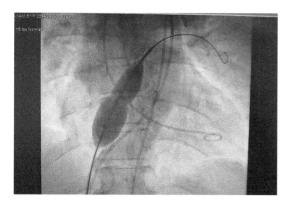

Figure 12.1 Temporary balloon-occlusion test using an Amplatzer sizing balloon.

is an increase in the risk of paradoxical embolism in pregnant patients with unrepaired ASDs or partially endothelialized ASD devices in situ. The existing pulmonary hypertension may worsen during the second or third trimester and may worsen right-heart failure in unoperated ASDs.

Limited studies have shown that obstetrical outcomes are similar in repaired and unrepaired ASDs. Closure of ASD is rarely required during pregnancy. But in selected cases where there is cyanosis due to right-to-left shunting, there may be risk of worsening heart failure without PAH, poor foetal growth or recurrent stroke after ASD closure. To minimize the risk to the developing foetus, when indicated, percutaneous ASD closure can be done in the second trimester with transesophageal and transthoracic echocardiogram with minimal fluoro guidance to reduce fluoro exposure to the growing foetus.[11] The rare case of surgical closure has been reported, but due to adverse effects of the cardiopulmonary bypass to the developing foetus, surgical ASD closure is to be avoided and delayed until after delivery.

ATRIAL ARRHYTHMIAS

In patients with ASDs, 8% are complicated by atrial arrhythmias, especially atrial flutter/atrial fibrillation. Older age at the time of intervention, large ASD causing right-heart dilatation and fibrosis and pulmonary arterial hypertension are some of the risk factors for the increase in incidence of atrial arrhythmias apart from thyroid or mitral valve diseases. Paroxysmal atrial flutter and fibrillation resolve after device closure, but surgical closure is associated with late-onset scar-related atrial arrhythmias.[6] Persistent atrial flutter or atrial fibrillation does not resolve. Preoperative atrial arrhythmia status is the strongest predictor of future arrhythmia incidence.[5]

PARADOXICAL EMBOLISM

Cerebrovascular accidents and some arterial emboli in younger patients are presumed to be due to paradoxical embolism due to right-to-left shunting across a patent foramen ovale or ostium secundum ASD. Numerous studies have shown relationship between stroke and paradoxical embolism after correction of reversible factors, and closure of ASD/PFO is a long-term benefit of stroke prevention. The proposed mechanism of stroke in patients with PFO/ASD is transient increase in right-sided pressure and subsequent right-to-left shunting, which cause paradoxical embolism of clots from venous circulation to enter arterial circulation, leading to stroke, gangrene etc. Closure of such PFO/ASD has shown benefits and long-term secondary prevention.

CONCLUSION

Transcatheter closure of ostium secundum ASD has become the default strategy of choice, but it still poses challenges and risks in patients with pulmonary hypertension, atrial arrhythmias, elderly individuals and diastolic heart failure situations. Adequate precaution and some modifications need to be done prior to subjecting these patients to transcatheter or surgical closure, weighing the risk and benefit on an individual basis.

REFERENCES

1. Campbell M. Natural history of atrial septal defect. *Br Heart J.* 1970; 32(6):820–6. doi: 10.1136/hrt.32.6.820. PMID: 5212356; PMCID: PMC487420.
2. Murphy JG, Gersh BJ, McGoon MD, Mair DD, Porter CJ, Ilstrup DM, McGoon DC, Puga FJ, Kirklin JW, Danielson GK. Long-term outcome after surgical repair of isolated atrial septal defect. Follow-up at 27 to 32 years. N Engl J Med. 1990 13; 323(24):1645–50. doi: 10.1056/NEJM199012133232401. PMID: 2233961.
3. Rao PS. When and how should atrial septal defects be closed in adults? *J Invasive Cardiol.* 2009; 21(2):76–82.
4. Humenberger M, Rosenhek R, Gabriel H, et al. Benefit of atrial septal defect closure in adults: Impact of age. *Eur Heart J.* 2011; 32(5):553–60.
5. Holzer R, Hijazi ZM. Interventional approach to congenital heart disease. Curr Opin Cardiol. 2004;19(2):84–90. PMID: 15075731.
6. Komar M, Olszowska M, Podolec P. The benefit of atrial septal defect closure in elderly patients. *Clin Interv Aging*, 2014; 9:1101–7.

7. Jategaonkar S, Scholtz W, Schmidt H, Horstkotte D. Percutaneous closure of atrial septal defects echocardiographic and functional results in patients older than 60 years. *Circ Cardiovasc Interv.* 2009; 2(2):85–9.

8. Balint OH, Samman A, Haberer K, Tobe L, McLaughlin P, Siu SC, Horlick E, Granton J, Silversides CK. Outcomes in patients with pulmonary hypertension undergoing percutaneous atrial septal defect closure. *Heart.* 2008;94(9):1189–93. doi: 10.1136/ hrt.2006.114660. Epub 2007 Oct 11. PMID: 17932093.

9. Miranda WR, Hagler DJ, Reeder GS, et al. Temporary balloon occlusion of atrial septal defects in suspected or documented left ventricular diastolic dysfunction: Hemodynamic and clinical findings. *Catheter Cardiovasc Interv.* 2019; 93(6):1069–75.

10. Yamamoto H, Shinke T, Otake H, et al. Investigation of hemodynamic changes during balloon occlusion test for percutaneous atrial septal defect closure. *J Am Coll Cardiol.* 2016; 67(13):935.

11. Zhang DZ, Zhu XY, Lv B, et al. Trial occlusion to assess the risk of persistent pulmonary arterial hypertension after closure of a large patent ductus arteriosus in adolescents and adults with elevated pulmonary artery pressure. *Circ Cardiovasc Interv.* 2014; 7(4):473–81.

12. Yong G, Khairy P, De Guise P, et al. Pulmonary arterial hypertension in patients with transcatheter closure of secundum atrial septal defects a longitudinal study. *Circ Cardiovasc Interv.* 2009; 2(5):455–62.

13. Bredy C, Mongeon FP, Leduc L, Dore A, Khairy P. Pregnancy in adults with repaired/ unrepaired atrial septal defect. *J Thorac Dis.* 2018; 10(Suppl 24):S2945–52.

14. Chiu SN, Wu MH, Tsai CT, et al. Atrial flutter/fibrillation in patients receiving transcatheter closure of atrial septal defect. *J Formos Med Association.* 2017; 116(7):522–8.

15. Taniguchi M, Akagi T, Ohtsuki S, et al. Transcatheter closure of atrial septal defect in elderly patients with permanent atrial fibrillation. *Catheter Cardiovasc Interv.* 2009; 73:682–686.

13

Newer frontiers in imaging: Three-dimensional (3D) echo and intracardiac echocardiography (ICE)

S J KABILAN, A A PILLAI

THREE-DIMENSIONAL (3D) ECHOCARDIOGRAM IN ATRIAL SEPTAL DEFECTS: CONCEPTS AND PROTOCOLS

The interatrial septum (IAS) is a complex, dynamic, three-dimensional anatomic structure A 2D echocardiogram cannot give a complete orientation of the atrial septal defects.[1] Two-dimensional imaging cannot align or interrogate the IAS because it does not exist in a true flat plane. Three-dimensional imaging with high frame rates and temporal resolution helps in defining the dynamic morphology of the defect, accurately determining atrial septal defect (ASD) size and shape and the relationship of ASD to the surrounding cardiac structures.[2]

At present, 3D matrix array transducers are composed of nearly 3000 individually connected and simultaneously active piezoelectric elements with frequencies ranging from 2 to 4 MHz and 5 to 7 MHz for transthoracic and transesophageal transducers, respectively. There are three different planes in which electronically controlled firing of elements in the matrix generates scan lines. They are x-axis or azimuthal direction; y-axis or axial direction and z-axis or vertical direction (elevation). And finally a volumetric pyramid of data is acquired. The image quality will be affected by point spread function of the system, which represents the imaging system response to a point input. The best images with less blurring will be obtained when using the axial dimension and more blurring while using the elevation dimension as the approximate spread in the axial (y) dimension is 0.5 mm and 3 mm in the elevation (z) dimension.[3]

In the parasternal approach, because the structures are primarily imaged in axial and lateral dimensions, good quality images are obtained. Poorer-quality images are obtained in the apical approach, which mostly uses the lateral and elevation dimensions.

The three different methods for 3D data set acquisition are (i) multiplane imaging, (ii) real-time live 3D imaging and (iii) multibeat electrocardiogram (ECG) gated imaging.[4] In multiplane mode, at a high frame rate, multiple 2D views can be acquired using predefined plane orientations. This is useful in situations like atrial fibrillation or interventricular dyssynchrony, where assessment of multiple views from same cardiac cycle is useful. In real-time mode, image orientation and plane can be changed by rotating or tilting the probe. Multibeat acquisition requires sequential acquisitions of narrow smaller volumes acquired from several ECG-gated cardiac cycles. Cropping, slicing and rotation were the three main actions done by the operator to obtain the desired view from a 3D volumetric dataset. Cropping is the process of removing irrelevant neighbouring tissue. Volume rendering, surface rendering and tomographic slices were the three different display modalities for depth perception of 3D images.[4]

The 3D echocardiogram has advantages in assessing size of the ASD in that it is radiation free compared to sizing-balloon measurement of ASD diameter and is non-invasive compared to TEE, which usually requires general anaesthesia in the paediatric population and carries the risk of aspiration and esophageal perforation.[5] Furthermore, 3D TTE has been shown to better approximate the dimensions and location and the anatomy of surrounding structures compared to 2D images. The American Society of Echocardiography currently recommends 2D TEE during percutaneous closure and repair of ASDs. But this is dependent on the observer's mental ability to recreate these images in 3D space, which can be difficult. But 3D imaging circumvents this problem by providing real-time three-dimensional images, aiding the operator in better assessment of ASDs and transcatheter closure.

Three-dimensional imaging of atrial septal defect is a potentially helpful tool in assessing the ASD device and its points of contact or pressure. For transthoracic 3D images, the subcostal view is the preferred view because its projection is en face to the atrial septum. In a prospective study, comparing 2D TTE, 2D TEE and 3D TTE in 37 patients with OS-ASD who underwent transcatheter device closure, there was significant correlation between the ASD diameter measured by 3D TTE and that by TEE ($r = 0.759$, $p - 0.001$).[6] Also, the rims of OS-ASD were assessed using 3D TEE, and atrioventricular rim (AV rim) was assessed in particular to avoid encroachment of the mitral valve and aorta. A cut-off value of 8.3 mm for AV rim was derived with an accuracy of 83.3% to avoid the encroachment on the aortico-mitral continuity plan than the previously published ratio ($1.5 \times$ ASD size). There was a direct relationship between the ratio of the left disc of the device to the total septum.[5] A new formula was constructed for device choice: ½ the defect size + AV rim length (not ≤ 8 mm) = ½ the left disc size of the device.

MORPHOLOGY OF ASD

OS-ASD will not be circular as assumed most of the time. It can be circular or oval or multiple fenestrations in the atrial septum maybe present. A 3D echocardiogram can be used to assess the various morphologies of atrial septal defects, such as oval or circular. A defect is considered oval when the ratio of the shortest diameter to the longest diameter ≤ 0.75, when measured using computed tomography.[7]

Also, the shape of the defect varies dynamically with different phases of cardiac cycle, which can be recorded with live 3D echocardiographic imaging. The maximum size of an ASD is seen in late ventricular systole and minimum size during late left ventricular diastole.[8]

3D TEE

In a study of patients undergoing 3D TEE, a protocol was developed for properly orienting the interatrial septum and ASDs.[9] The horizontal axis runs from right to left edge of the screen, the vertical axis from top to bottom of the screen and the z-axis is perpendicular to the computer monitor. The lateral (azimuth) direction is encoded in red, the elevation direction in green and the depth direction in blue by convention. Three-dimensional TEE images were obtained in the following modalities: (i) biplane imaging (a side-by-side display of a pair of 2D TEE images that are 90 degrees apart), (ii) full-volume imaging, (iii) narrow-angle live 3D imaging and (iv) wide-angle 3D zoom imaging. The image acquisitions at 0 degree and 90 degrees are performed first.

IMAGE ACQUISITION AT 0 DEGREE (TUPLE MANOEUVRE)

The 3D zoom mode is selected after getting a good midesophageal view of the interatrial septum at 0 degree in 2D mode. In the initial pair of biplane images appearing on the screen, the left image

TUPLE (tilt-up-then-left) maneuver

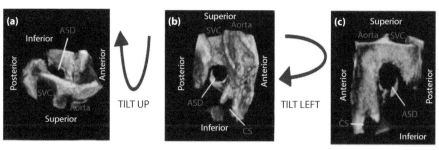

Figure 13.1 Image acquisition with TUPLE manoeuvre. (Adapted from Saric et al. *Journal of American Society of Echocardiography*, 2010.)[10]

shows the lateral (azimuth, or red) plane and the right image shows the elevation (green) plane. There is a region-of-interest selection box in each image, and by moving it up and down the screen, the user can determine which portion of the depth (blue) plane will be displayed in the subsequent 3D view. After selecting the region of interest, a 3D zoom view is obtained and the interatrial septum appears in its long axis view, which is referred to as the 'opening scene'. This view is then manipulated to get an en face view of the interatrial septum, which is the view as a surgeon would view it. In the tilt-up-then-left (TUPLE) manoeuvre, an initial 3D image of IAS is first tilted up along its horizontal axis to reveal en face view from right atrial perspective. The superior vena cava (SVC) and aorta are the most important structures in this view. The SVC is at the top of the screen and aortic valve and ascending aorta are on the right of the screen. In the next step, the image is tilted left around the vertical axis by 180 degrees to obtain the en face

view of IAS from the left atrial perspective. Here the superior rim is at the top of the screen, the aortic rim on left side and the ostia of pulmonary veins on the right side of the monitor (Figure 13.1).

IMAGE ACQUISITION (TUPLE PLUS ROTATE LEFT IN Z-AXIS [ROLZ] MANOEUVRE)

As obtained previously, the opening scene 3D zoom image is obtained at 90 degrees. This has the same orientation as the bicaval view in 2D TEE. The image is tilted up to reveal the right atrial side of the septum in the first step, and the SVC now appears on the right side of the screen. Then, to obtain view of the IAS from left atrial side, it has to be rotated by 90 degrees in counterclockwise direction in the z-axis.

Three-dimensional TEE helps in assessing the rims of the ASD in a well-delineated manner (Figure 13.2). Three-dimensional TEE is a valuable

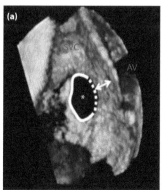
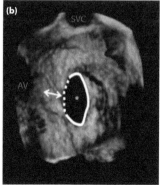

Figure 13.2 3D TEE showing rims of OS-ASD from right atrial side (a) and left atrial side (b). (Adapted from Saric et al. *Journal of American Society of Echocardiography*, 2010.)[10]

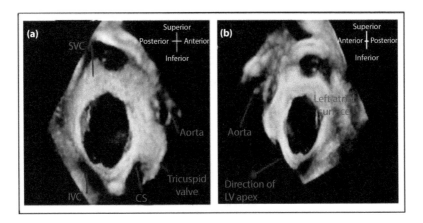

Figure 13.3 3D TEE views of OS-ASD from right atrial view (a) and left atrial view (b). (Adapted from Pushparajah et al. *JACC: Cardiovascular Imaging*, September 2010.)[11]

tool in visualizing an OS ASD and its anatomical orientation to its neighbouring vital structures. The OS-ASD seen through the right atrial as well as left atrial side is depicted in Figure 13.3. Also, rare types of atrial septal defects with multiple fenestrations which are difficult to visualize in 2D TEE can be identified using a 3D TEE (Figure 13.4). Atrial septal defects like coronary sinus ASD, either SVC or IVC type could be easily recognized using a 3D TEE (Figure 13.5).

Three-dimensional TEE helps to determine whether sufficient tissue rim is caught between the two plates of the device.[11]

In a prospective study of 30 children (mean age 9.8 ± 2.8 years, median weight 26.5 kg) who underwent percutaneous device closure of ASD, 2D TEE, 3D TEE and balloon sizing were compared

in assessing the ASD shape, diameter and area.[6] In this study, all children underwent TTE for initial assessment of ASD and rims. Patients with deficient rims except the aortic rim and those weighing <18 kg were not included. The procedure was done under general anaesthesia. Pre-procedural 2D TEE was done initially to assess size and rims, followed by acquisition of 3D images in a real-time mode. The 2D TEE measurements and only the shape of ASD by 3D TEE en face view were available to the interventionist during the procedure. The rest of the 3D TEE measurements and analysis were done post-procedure offline independently after blinded for 2D TEE measurements, balloon sizing and device size. There was no statistically significant difference in ASD diameter between 2D and 3D TEE. There was significant correlation between

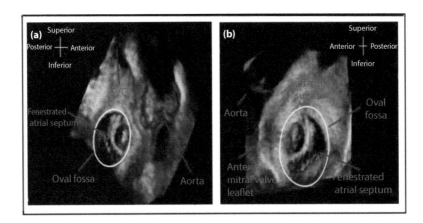

Figure 13.4 3D TEE showing fenestrated ASDs from right atrial view (a) and left atrial view (b). (Adapted from Pushparajah et al. *JACC: Cardiovascular Imaging*, September 2010.)[11]

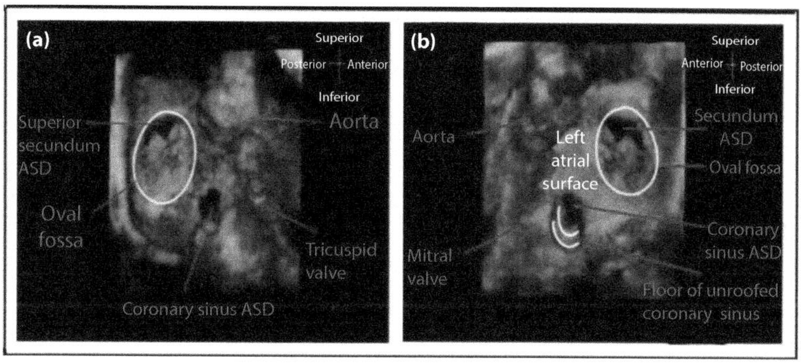

Figure 13.5 3D TEE showing coronary sinus ASD and a superior OS-ASD from right atrial view (a) and left atrial view (b). (Adapted from Pushparajah et al. *JACC: Cardiovascular Imaging*, September 2010.)[11]

the balloon sizing with ASD diameter by 2D and 3D TEE, even though the balloon-sized diameter was the largest. The shape of the ASD was oval in 47.7% of the patients. There was a greater difference between BS and maximum 3D TEE diameters in round ASDs than in oval ASDs. The difference in diameter between maximal diameters by 3D TEE and 2D TEE was higher in oval ASDs than round ASDs.[8,12]

In this study for predicting the balloon sizing of the defect they have suggested a prediction model. If the shape of ASD is oval and maximal diameter by 3D TEE is ≤21 mm, balloon sizing is predicted by adding 1 mm to the 3D TEE maximal diameter and adding 2 mm if the oval ASD is more than 21 mm. If the shape is round in the 3D en face view, balloon sizing is predicted by adding 4 mm to the maximal 3D TEE diameter of ASD if size is ≤21 mm and by adding 5 mm if the size is greater than 21 mm. The ASD diameters measured by balloon sizing are overestimated compared with 3D TEE, particularly in round ASDs.[6,12]

A study was conducted to assess the incremental value of unenhanced real-time 3D TEE over contrast TTE, in comparison with contrast TEE in detection of PFO in patients with migraine headache or unexplained cerebrovascular ischemic events. Overall, the diagnostic accuracy of RT-3D TTE was greater than contrast TTE (sensitivity 83% vs. 44%, specificity 100% vs. 100%, NPV of 88% vs. 69%). But for PFO effect size < 2 mm, the sensitivity was lower (76%) compared with gold standard contrast TEE.[3] The limitations of 3D TEE were due to its larger size; it was suitable for patients weighing more than 20 kg, and 3D full-volume

mode was prone to stitch artefacts.[12] In a study of patients with OS-ASD, it was reported that 2D TEE images were superior in spatial and time resolution compared with RT 3D TEE images.[13] In cases of ostium primum ASDs, 3D echocardiogram could provide a better assessment of cleft mitral valve. The volumetric information of dilated RV and geometric details of dilated tricuspid annulus in en face view in 3D echo could be used for tricuspid annuloplasty during ASD patch closure.[13] There was a strong negative correlation between 3D echocardiogram-derived RV ejection fraction and RV afterload. For closure of multiple ASDs, a 3D echo X-ray navigation system can be useful in which TEE and fluoroscopic images are integrated, permitting the identification of shape and location of ASDs evaluated by 3D TEE on fluoroscopy.

INTRACARDIAC ECHOCARDIOGRAPHY (ICE): USE IN DIAGNOSIS AND TREATMENT

Protocol

Intracardiac echocardiography is an excellent tool to assess the ASD size and rims and for guiding transcatheter closure.[14] It has the advantage of better visualization of posterior/inferior atrial septum without requiring general anaesthesia or deep sedation. It also allows the operator to have complete control over image acquisition as a sonographer to do a TEE may not be required. The commonly used ICE catheter is AcuNav catheter (Biosense Webster, Inc., Diamond Bar, CA), which is a 64-element phase array catheter with frequencies between 5 and 19 MHz.[15] There are three knobs on the handle of the catheter for imaging in different planes. The top knob controls the anterior (clockwise) or posterior (counter clockwise) tilt; the middle knob controls the left (counter clockwise) and right (clockwise) tilts. The catheter is in neutral (straight) position when all the notches on the knobs are lined up. All the positions mentioned previously (anterior, posterior, right, left) apply only when all the notches are pointing anteriorly in a neutral position. When viewed from the feet looking towards the head, with the patient lying in supine position, a clock face should be imagined: 12 o'clock is straight anterior; 6 o'clock is straight posterior; 3 o'clock is straight left and 9 o'clock is straight right. The catheter should be kept as straight as possible, and the operator should hold the handle with the right hand and hold the shaft of the catheter next to the venous sheath with the left hand (Figure 13.6).

The catheter should be advanced through the left femoral venous approach into the low right atrium. The home view is when the notches are neutral, with the catheter at the 1 o'clock or 2 o'clock position.[16] The structures visualized in this view are Eustachian valve, tricuspid valve and RV inflow. Colour flow Doppler can be used to assess the tricuspid regurgitation.

A biventricular outflow view is made by rotating the catheter half past 2 o'clock to the 3 o'clock position. The left ventricular long axis, aorta and pulmonary artery can be visualized in this view. From the outflow view, on further rotation of the catheter to the 4 o' clock position, the atrial septum above the coronary sinus can be visualized, along

with mitral valve and left atrial appendage. So this view can be used to assess whether the ASD septal occlude is impinging on the mitral valve, causing mitral regurgitation.

If the catheter is further rotated in clockwise direction between the 4 o'clock and 5 o'clock positions, the left superior and inferior pulmonary veins can be visualized entering the posterior aspect of the left atrium. In this position colour flow can be used to assess the pulmonary venous blood flow also. After bringing the catheter to the neutral position in the left pulmonary vein view, it should be locked by rotating the bottom knob counterclockwise. At this point, if the top knob is rotated counterclockwise, the atrial septum can be visualized, along with the aorta on the short-axis view, and the aortic rim can be interrogated here. The catheter should be pulled inferiorly to visualize the posterior inferior portion of interatrial septum. In the short-axis view the handle should be fixed in position and the middle knob should be closely rotated. Now the superior vena cava will be visualized, along with the superior aspect of the interatrial septum. On continued clockwise rotation, the inferior vena cava and the posterior portion of the septum can also be seen, along with a portion of right pulmonary veins. To visualize the mitral valve, the catheter should be first brought back to home view so that the tricuspid valve is visualized. Further clockwise rotation allows visualization of the anterior mitral leaflet in 7 o'clock to 8 o'clock position. So during device deployment, the relationship between the device and mitral valve can be ascertained in this view.

The commercially available ICE catheter systems are 8-F AcuNav catheter, and 9-F ViewFlex-Plus (St. Jude Medical, St. Paul, USA). The 10-F AcuNav catheter carries a matrix transducer, providing a 22 degrees × 90 degrees real-time volume image from cardiac chambers or neighbouring vessels.[17] Beyond the assessment of ASD rims, ICE also helps in guiding device closure. During device deployment, the ICE also depicts the release of the left-side disc, which opens inside the left atrium near the mouth of the pulmonary vein. It will also show how well the left atrial disc is approximated against the inter atrial septum. While the delivery cable is under traction, the ICE also demonstrates the release of the right-sided disc inside the RA, and the left sided disc remaining on the left side was lined up with the interatrial septum. ICE

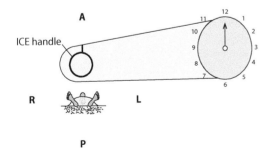

Figure 13.6 Patient representation as viewed from foot of bed. The ICE handle is demonstrated with notches on handle pointing anteriorly, and rotation of catheter is referenced to clock face.[15] (Illustration by Saranya Gousy.)

provides better image resolution than TEE, particularly when complications develop.[8]

For younger patients of reproductive age undergoing device closure for ASD, ICE helps in reducing the fluoroscopic time, thereby reducing the radiation exposure. It is also helpful in paediatric patients with ASD undergoing device closure by avoiding the potential esophageal injury due to insertion of TEE probe. This is particularly helpful in transcatheter closure of multiple fenestrated defects requiring simultaneous device deployments. The major advantage of RT-3D TEE compared to 2D ICE or conventional TEE is the ability to demonstrate the dynamic morphology of atrial septal defects such as elliptical, oblong or fenestrated shapes.[18] The three-dimensional zoom mode is highly useful for observing the position of guidewires, sheaths and devices in real time. Real-time 3D ICE catheters such as 10-F AcuNav were also developed, but the main limitation for this approach is small image volume in the near field.

In a study of 60 patients, interatrial communication (40 ASD, 20 PFO) and ICE-guided device closure was done. Apart from sizing the defect, it also revealed a Chiari network with thrombus in one patient and additional septal defects in four patients, which were not seen with TEE. For defects located in the inferior part of the interatrial septum, ICE is superior to TEE for aspects of visualization. Despite viewing the septum from different angles, ICE does allow for multiplane imaging. There is also a rare complication of vascular injury caused by placing a 8-F sheath for ICE catheter access.[15] One retrospective study analyzed 52 patients who underwent transcatheter closure of ASD under ICE guidance without requirement of general anaesthesia or TEE. Only three patients had paroxysmal atrial fibrillation post-procedure, which was resolved with treatment. Also they did not use the sizing balloon here as the ICE catheter was solely used for assessing size of the defect and rims and confirming the position before deployment. Compared with the baseline TEE before the procedure, which measured a mean defect size of 18.1 mm, the mean diameter measured by ICE was slightly larger (i.e., 20.2 mm).

Data on device closure with ICE guidance in the paediatric population are lacking. There is one retrospective study in which the mean age of 115 patients who underwent transcatheter device closure was 12 ± 6 years. About 34% of the population underwent cardiac catheterization and ICE without requirement of general anaesthesia. ICE had a good correlation with the preprocedural TTE. The mean fluoroscopy time was 21 ± 10 minutes. In spite of the correlation of ASD size between ICE and TTE, TTE underestimated static defect size relative to ICE. The atrial septal anatomy was appreciated well with ICE so that it identified deficiencies of critical rims or multiple ASDs that were missed out in TTE in six patients.[14]

Another retrospective study analyzed 46 patients, 50% of whom underwent TEE-guided closure and the remaining 50% underwent ICE-guided closure of the atrial septal defect. Fluoroscopy time and procedure time were significantly lower in the ICE-guided closure group compared to the TEE group.

The success rates of transcatheter closure of atrial septal defects have improved dramatically due to the advances in imaging techniques. Advanced imaging modalities like 3D TEE and ICE help in better visualization of the ASD, its rims, morphology, sizing of the device and feasibility for device closure. Also intraprocedural imaging guidance is invaluable for positioning the device properly before deployment. Newer imaging modalities pave a better way for the development of techniques and devices for successful closure of anatomically challenging atrial septal defects.

REFERENCES

1. Vaidyanathan B, Simpson JM, Kumar RK. Transesophageal echocardiography for device closure of atrial septal defects: Case selection, planning, and procedural guidance. *JACC Cardiovasc Imaging*. 2009; 2: 1238–42.

2. Hascoet S, Hadeed K, Marchal P, Dulac Y, Alacoque X, Heitz F, Acar P. The relation between atrial septal defect shape, diameter, and area using three-dimensional transoesophageal echocardiography and balloon sizing during percutaneous closure in children. *Eur Heart J: Cardiovasc Imaging*. 2015; 16:747–55.

3. Monte I, Grasso S, Licciardi S, Badano LP. Head-to-head comparison of real-time three-dimensional transthoracic echocardiography with transthoracic and transesophageal two-dimensional

echocardiography for the detection of patent foramen ovale. *Eur J Echocardiogr.* 2010; 11:245–49.

4. Price MJ, Smith MR, Rubenson DS. Utility of on-line three-dimensional transesophageal echocardiography during percutaneous atrial septal defect closure. *Catheter Cardiovasc Interv* 2010; 75:570–7.

5. Huang X, Shen J, Huang Y, et al. En face view of atrial septal defect by two-dimensional transthoracic echocardiography: Comparison to real-time three dimensional transesophageal echocardiography. *J Am Soc Echocardiogr.* July 2010; 23(7):714–2.

6. El-Saiedi SA, Agha HM, Shaltoot MF, et al. ASD device closure in pediatrics: 3-dimensional transthoracic echocardiography perspective. *J Saudi Heart Assoc.* 2018; 30(3): 188–97.

7. Song J, Lee SY, Baek JS, Shim WS, Choi EY. Outcome of transcatheter closure of oval shaped atrial septal defect with amplatzer septal occluder. *Yonsei Med J.* 2013; 54(5): 1104–1109.

8. Su C-H, Weng KP, Chang JK, et al. Assessment of atrial septal defect role of real-time 3D color Doppler echocardiography for interventional catheterization. *Acta Cardiol Sin.* 2005; 21:146–52.

9. Seo JS, Song JM, Kim YH, et al. Effect of atrial septal defect shape evaluated using three-dimensional transesophageal echocardiography on size measurements for percutaneous closure. *J Am Soc Echocardiography.* 2012; 25:1031–40.

10. Saric M, Perk G, Purgess JR, Kronzon I. Imaging atrial septal defects by real-time 3D transesophageal echocardiography: Step by step approach. *J Am Soc Echocardiogr,* 2010; 23(11):1128–35.

11. Pusparajah K, Miller O, Simpson J. 3D echo-cardiography of the atrial septum. *JACC: Cardiovasc Imaging,* 2010; 3(9):981–4.

12. Lang R, Goldstein SA, Kronzon I, Khandheria BK, Mon-Ani V. *ASE's comprehensive echocardiography.* 2nd ed. Philadelphia (PA): Elsevier; 2016.

13. Yang HS. Three-dimensional echocardiography in adult congenital heart disease. *Korean J Intern Med.* 2017; 32:577–88.

14. Zanchetta M, Onorato E, Rigatelli G, et al. Intracardiac echocardiography-guided trans catheter closure of secundum atrial septal defect: A new efficient device selection method. *J Am Coll Cardiol.* 2003; 42: 1677–82.

15. Balzer D. Intracardiac echocardiographic atrial septal defect closure. *Methodist Debakey Cardiovasc J.* 2014; 10(2):88–92.

16. Luxenberg DM, Silvestry FE, Herrmann HC, Cao Q-L, Rohatgi S, Hijazi ZM. Use of a new 8 French intracardiac echocardiographic catheter to guide device closure of atrial septal defects and patent foramen ovale in small children and adults: Initial clinical experience. *J Invasive Cardiol.* 2005; 17: 540–5.

17. Bartel T, Mueller S. Device closure of inter-atrial communications: Peri-interventional echocardiographic assessment. *Eur Heart J Cardiovasc Imaging.* 2013; 14:618–24.

18. Boccalandro F, Baptista E, Muench A, Carter C, Smalling RW. Comparison of intracardiac echocardiography versus trans-esophageal echocardiography guidance for percutaneous trans catheter closure of atrial septal defect. *Am J Cardiol.* 2004; 93: 437–40.

Index

Italicized and **bold** pages refer to figures and tables respectively